W9-AHB-793

This practical guide is easily readable and well-organized. Cara Novy-Bennewitz, a breast cancer survivor herself, provides readers with a comprehensive strategy that goes well beyond basic treatment information. I highly recommend **Diagnosis: Breast Cancer** *to anyone seeking empowerment on their breast cancer journey.*

~**Patrick Maguire, M.D.**
Coastal Carolina Radiation Oncology

I absolutely love this text! It fills a major gap in critically important breast cancer patient knowledge. The personalized forms and questions for healthcare workers are of extreme value. Congratulations for creating an extremely useful resource for the breast cancer patients and their families.

~**David S. Alberts, M.D.**
Director, University of Arizona Cancer Center

When you hear you have cancer, one of the first questions is always: what do I do now? Unfortunately you learn very quickly that there is no "answer book." You must gather all of your options, you must decide. Finally there is a tool to help you. **Diagnosis: Breast Cancer** *is that tool. It provides everything that you will need, and it is all delivered in an understanding and loving manner so you feel supported as you move through this journey. Thank you, Cara. I wish I had had this book when I was diagnosed!*

~**Peggy Devine**
Founder & President
Cancer Information & Support Network, Inc.

At the most vulnerable time in your life, your cancer diagnosis, you will be asked to participate in decision making that will impact all aspects of your life. The complexities of the decisions to be made, the concepts to grasp, and even the language of medicine are overwhelming. **Diagnosis: Breast Cancer** *will allow you to organize and simplify the complexities of breast cancer diagnosis, treatment, and survivorship. Cara's experience as both patient and educator are translated into a wonderfully-crafted working book which will aid the newly-diagnosed patient in making the most appropriate decisions for herself. I recommend this book to all newly diagnosed breast cancer patients.*

~**Richard M. Boulay, M.D.**
Gynecological Oncology,Obstetrics & Gynecology.
Journeythroughcancer.com

Cara Novy-Bennewitz provides a very practical guidebook for those patients newly diagnosed with breast cancer. She discusses the basics of breast cancer diagnosis and treatment, including surgery, radiation therapy, and chemotherapy/hormonal therapy. In addition, worksheets are provided to help keep the patient and her support team organized and to ensure that important questions get asked. This book should be very helpful for someone newly diagnosed with breast cancer, as well as her friends and family members.

~**Deanna J. Attai, M.D., F.A.C.S.**
Center For Breast Care, Inc.
Member, Board of Directors and Chair,
Communications Committee—American Society of Breast Surgeons
Fellow, American College of Surgeons

Diagnosis: Breast Cancer *is a wonderful resource for those newly diagnosed with breast cancer. It is easy to read and to understand with helpful visuals throughout the book. The worksheets are extremely useful during an incredibly overwhelming time. It helps the reader organize their thoughts and to formulate a step-by-step action plan by giving them tools. There are many breast cancer books, but this one takes out the guess work. It is a one-stop shop book that I would recommend to anyone that was just diagnosed with breast cancer!*

~**Runi Limary**
Senior Certified Patient Navigator/Young Survivor Services
Breast Cancer Resource Center, Austin, TX

Cara's true gift is sharing knowledge and tips as a breast cancer survivor. The book is straight-forward, non-intimidating, and made easy to understand from start to finish. An essential guide for any woman after breast cancer diagnosis!

~**Jonny Imerman**
Testicular Cancer Survivor (2x)
Chief Mission Officer, IMERMAN ANGELS

When the doctor tells you that you have breast cancer, your critical-thinking and organizational skills can fly out the window. **Diagnosis: Breast Cancer** *can help you. Cara Novy-Bennewitz has crafted an invaluable resource for newly diagnosed breast cancer patients and their families. From diagnosis through treatment, and into survivorship,* **Diagnosis: Breast Cancer** *is your ally and companion. It is filled with factual information, explained in easy-to-understand terms.*

The myriads of charts are available to help you organize and track your information and treatment. Helpful tips, clear illustrations, questions for doctors, worksheets, and logs are found throughout the workbook. First-hand advice from breast cancer survivors graces the pages of this book, along with many inspirational quotes. The Glossary and Internet Resources sections are comprehensive as well. **Diagnosis: Breast Cancer** *will be an invaluable tool for patients and their caregivers as they find their way through breast cancer! I cannot think of a better resource and companion for breast cancer patients as they navigate the road through cancer-land!*

~**Bethany Aronow, M.A., L.P.C.**
Cancer Counselor & Survivor

Windy City Publishers
2118 Plum Grove Rd., #349
Rolling Meadows, IL 60008
www.windycitypublishers.com

Published in the United States of America

10 9 8 7 6 5 4 3 2 1

First Edition: 2012

Library of Congress Control Number: 2011945010

ISBN: 978-1-935766-17-9

Cover Production by Amanda Inkinen
Medical Illustrations by Jeremy Brotherton

Windy City Publishers
Chicago

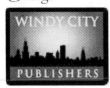

Diagnosis: Breast Cancer

The Best Action Plan for Navigating Your Journey

CARA NOVY-BENNEWITZ

Dedication

This book is dedicated to my loving husband Kirk, my amazing son Kilmer, and to my family, whose love and support mean the world to me.

Acknowledgements

I would like to acknowledge my incredible treatment team and the medical experts who provided me with outstanding care and generously donated their time and energy to ensure the information provided here is accurate.

Surgical Oncology: Katharine Yao, M.D., F.A.C.S., Clinical Assistant Professor, NorthShore University HealthSystem

Medical Oncology: Douglas Merkel, M.D., Clinical Assistant Professor, NorthShore University HealthSystem

Plastic Surgery: Michael Howard, M.D., Clinical Assistant Professor, University of Chicago, Pritzker School of Medicine, Division of Plastic Surgery, NorthShore University HealthSystem

Radiation Oncology: Arif Y. Shaikh, M.D., Clinical Instructor of Radiation Oncology, NorthShore University Health System, and William Bloomer, MD, NorthShore University HealthSystem

Oncology Nurses: Bonnie Ryszka, RN, BSN, Collaborative Practice Nurse and Debbie Nechi-Fragassi, RN, BSN, OCN Collaborative Practice Nurse, NorthShore University HealthSystem

Genetics: Scott M. Weissman, MS, LCG, NorthShore University Health ystem

Oncology Nurse Navigator: Beth Weigel, RN, NorthShore University HealthSystem

I would also like to acknowledge my fellow cancer travelers Joyce B., Sue B., Bette H., Judy H., Holly H., Frances M., and Cindy S. for their willingness to share valuable insights and personal experiences from the trenches.

A special thank you goes to Lise Marinelli, Kristyn Friske, and Janet Dooley at Windy City Publishers, who made the process of writing this book a delight. Finally, thank you to Jeremy Brotherton for providing wonderful medical illustrations.

Foreword
by Kathy Yao, M.D., F.A.C.S.

It is during our darkest moments that we must focus to see the light.

-Aristotle Onassis

I have diagnosed many breast cancer patients throughout my career. It is the least favorite part of what I do, especially when I see the fear and angst they feel when they hear my words. Many times it's the worst news they have ever heard and the "unknowns" can easily outweigh what they have, or will, read about their upcoming journey. The loss of control, in any situation, is a breeding ground for chaos, fear, and confusion—never a good place to start.

Telling a patient "not to worry" may be a brief moment of comfort for them. But they are easily forgotten words, especially outside the relative safety of a doctor's office. But if I can throw them a lifeline, a guidebook, that can help alleviate the anxiety, I have given them the best start for navigating their way to recovery. This book was written to take the fear out of those initial moments and to guide the newly diagnosed patients through a sea of information.

Breast cancer is a heterogeneous disease. This means there are many types of cancer, so it's important to focus on your case and not on your friend's or neighbor's. In addition, tumor size and node status are not the only things that determine prognosis. Fortunately, we have treatments for all sorts of cancers. Through many years of research, we have developed "targeted" therapies, directed at specific types of breast cancer. This once deadly disease is treatable and has one of the best survival rates of any of the cancers out there—the advances in treatments are truly amazing and have come far, especially in the past ten years.

Your support system can be a key factor in aiding your recovery—don't be afraid to use it. Your friends and family want to help so let them. Staying as calm and composed as you can, maintaining physical and emotional balance and actively participating in your treatment decisions will all help reduce the stress you will certainly be feeling. This book will help you achieve these goals and give you a sense of control over your cancer.

Cara has written this book not only from a breast cancer patient perspective but from that of an educator as well. She has taken an incredibly complex subject and consolidated and organized the information into an easy-to-use format. This guide is meant to "de-stress" the breast cancer journey and empower the patient. I truly commend her work. On behalf of all the newly diagnosed breast cancer patients out there, Cara, I thank you.

Kathy Yao, M.D.

Kathy Yao is Director of the Breast Surgical Program at NorthShore University HealthSystem and a Clinical Associate Professor of the University of Chicago, Pritzker School of Medicine. She completed a surgical residency at Northwestern University in Chicago and then went on to a two-year surgical oncology fellowship at the John Wayne Cancer Institute in California. Prior to the NorthShore position, she was Director of the Breast Clinical Program at Loyola University Medical Center. She has devoted her practice to disease of the breast.

Table of Contents

> *Do not let what you*
> *cannot do interfere*
> *with what you can.*
>
> **- John Wooden**

Introduction

When my doctor told me I had cancer, all I could think was: *Really*??

I was under the impression that I could prevent cancer. I was completely dedicated to staying healthy. I worked out. I didn't drink. I didn't smoke. In fact, I was a personal trainer and physical educator. And still I got cancer. While there are many things we can do to prevent certain illnesses, there are no guarantees that we won't get sick.

If you have recently been diagnosed with breast cancer or someone you care about has been diagnosed, you are probably experiencing a wide range of emotions including shock, fear, and even anger. I know I was.

My reaction was to quickly find as much information as I could. I knew that breast cancer had excellent recovery rates, but I needed a game plan. I hit bookstores and the Internet and immediately got overwhelmed. How can anyone sort through and absorb all this information? I couldn't. You can't. More importantly, you don't have to.

Once I slowed down and caught my breath, I realized I needed to approach my diagnosis in the same way I manage other areas of my life. In one of my favorite books, *The Success Principles*, Jack Canfield suggests defining your goal then "chunking it down" into smaller manageable steps. So that's what I did. The process instantly became more manageable.

I didn't want to get sidetracked online, wasting my valuable time reading about stuff that didn't apply to me. So I went to my doctors for advice on where I should look and what I should be looking for. With their help, once I knew the type of cancer I was facing, I was able to break down my treatment plan into manageable steps. So can you.

Like most successful projects, this book was a team effort involving many cancer specialists and fellow breast cancer survivors. There are many things in life you can't control. This book will help you with the ones you can.

—Cara

P.S. If you're looking for additional books to read, these three are a great balance between practical advice and in-depth medical information.

The 10 Best Questions for Surviving Breast Cancer
by Dede Bonner, Ph.D.
This book offers an in-depth explanation of the questions you should ask and why you should ask them.

Just Get Me Through This: A Practical Guide to Coping with Breast Cancer
by Deborah A. Cohen and Robert M. Gelfand
Although this book is geared toward readers with early stage breast cancer, it gives practical advice and tips for every phase of the journey.

Dr. Susan Love's Breast Book
by Susan Love, M.D.
It's pretty academic, but this is one of the top-rated comprehensive books on breast cancer.

How to Use This Book

Diagnosis: Breast Cancer is a worksheet-driven book designed to empower you and your loved ones while you navigate your journey from diagnosis to recovery. Each informational chapter is followed by a series of corresponding worksheets to help you make carefully considered decisions, stay organized, and remain proactive in your treatment choices. They help you answer who, what, where, and why and are meant to be written on, photocopied, or torn out.

Skip around, using only the chapters and worksheets that you need. Some will apply to you and some won't—it all depends on you and your treatment choices. Review worksheets before appointments and feel free to add you own questions or concerns.

**Additional copies are available online at *www.workingoutcancer.com*.
Just enter the word "navigate."**

This book is divided into three easy-to-use sections.

Part I: Getting Organized

Before heading into any battle you want to make sure you have excellent leadership that you trust and that you know what you are facing. This section has useful tips and information on how to surround yourself with strong allies, understand your diagnosis, and stay organized.

Part II: Treatment Information

When troops land in a foreign country, they often have to quickly pick up the native language to familiarize themselves with their surroundings. That's what this section is about. Each chapter includes a brief overview of some treatment options you could be facing and helps you to gather your information step by step. This section is not designed to teach you everything about breast cancer or to replace any medical advice. Read what you need and leave the rest.

Part III: Additional Resources

When gathering information it's vital to trust your sources. This section provides you with a directory of well-established, reputable Internet resources for gathering more information. A short glossary of common cancer terminology is also provided here.

Understanding the Worksheet Icons

Icons are designed to help you identify different types of worksheets. Below is a key to understanding the icons:

This icon alerts you to helpful Record Keeping worksheets. These sheets will help you document your medical and treatment information.

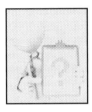

This icon alerts you to Questions for the Treatment Team. It's not uncommon to have a ton of questions, only to forget them as soon as you're with the doctor. These worksheets help you to remain focused.

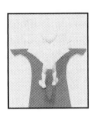

This icon alerts you to Medical Options and Opinions worksheets. You are going to be presented with different opinions and treatment options. These worksheets will help you weigh the advantages and disadvantages of each choice.

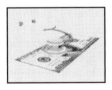

This icon alerts you to Medical and Insurance Expense worksheets. These worksheets will assist you in tracking all of your expenses associated with your breast cancer care.

Since this workbook is accessible to others, it's not meant to be a personal diary. Although you may record treatment information in this book, do not record sensitive financial information (such as social security numbers or bank account numbers) here.

Part I
Getting Organized

Where do you start when your goal is to beat breast cancer? With the first step. This section identifies some of the pre-treatment issues you may face and tells you what you can do now to help you through treatments.

- **Chapter 1** offers practical advice on getting organized and gathering information.

- **Chapter 2** explains breast cancer and additional diagnostic tests.

- **Chapter 3** helps you understand your pathology report.

- **Chapter 4** discusses how to gather and use support systems.

- **Chapter 5** offers practical advice on managing your day-to-day matters.

Worksheets Quick Reference Guide

You don't have to see
the whole staircase,
just take the first step.

- Martin Luther King

chapter

1

Gathering Your Tools

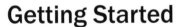

Getting Started

Learning you have cancer can feel like getting the wind knocked out of you. But once the initial shock, pain, and surprise subside, you can take action. Although you may want to "get rid of it" as quickly as possible, you don't have to rush or panic. Allow yourself time to sort through your emotions. Acknowledge your feelings, express them, and keep moving forward.

Creating Storage Systems

If you don't check your e-mail for a few days, that full inbox can feel overwhelming. The paperwork associated with cancer accumulates quickly and can make you feel the same way. Having cancer is stressful enough without the added burden of tracking all your bills and paperwork.

As you start gathering information, test results, and paperwork, you will need a place to put it all. Lower your stress and keep a handle on your documents by purchasing the following items:

❑ Expandable file folder or notebook (the American Cancer Society, *www.cancer.org*, and the Young Survival Coalition, *www.youngsurvival.org*, both provide these free of charge)

❑ Color-coded folders and markers

❑ Flash drive or backup drive for electronic records

❑ Journal or notebook for your personal thoughts and reflections

> The diagnosis of cancer is a deep shock, with much uncertainty. The more we gather information leading to a treatment plan, the more control we regain. A plan translates to less uncertainty. Keeping the multitude of information organized and at the ready is essential to managing the avalanche of details and emotions that accompany cancer treatment and return to wellness.
> —Frances M.

To stay organized:

- Create a separate file for each topic (lab reports, bills, insurance, etc.).

- Ask for copies of your test results, lab work, and reports.

- Address paperwork as you receive it.

- Record bill payments as they occur, not later.

- Keep all your material in one place.

The *Document Storage Worksheet* on page 40 helps you locate other personal documents if the need should arise. If you are having trouble getting organized, ask a friend or family member to help you. It's a good opportunity to take someone up on their offer to help. Your friends want to be of use.

What to Bring to Your Appointments

Make your appointments as informative and stress-free as possible by bringing:

❑ **A recording device:** Ask your doctors for permission to record your appointments. This is not unusual. This way you can review the information they give you to help you make informed decisions. Check to see if your cell phone has recording capability.

❑ **A capable companion:** Bring someone you can rely on to be a second set of eyes and ears. You probably will not process all the information you receive the first time you hear it.

❑ *Diagnosis: Breast Cancer*

❑ **Pathology reports, tests, and lab results**

❑ **Your insurance card and photo identification**

❑ **Pen and paper**

Remember that breast cancer is usually a very treatable disease.

Whom Do You See First?

One of the hardest parts of dealing with your diagnosis is figuring out what to do next. Start by asking the person who diagnosed your cancer who he or she thinks you should see first to learn more about your type of cancer. Some of the specialists who may be on your treatment team include:

- **Surgical Oncologist:** A surgeon who specializes in cancer. This person is usually the initial "team leader" in your treatment plan. Your breast surgeon will be responsible for surgically removing your tumor.

- **Pathologist:** This person is extremely important since he or she performs many tests on your tissue to determine the type, extent, and aggressiveness of your cancer. Make sure your pathologist specializes in breast cancer.

- **Plastic Surgeon:** This surgeon will perform your reconstructive surgery if you choose to pursue it.

- **Medical Oncologist:** a doctor specializing in a wide variety of treatments including chemical, hormonal, and biological therapies.

- **Oncology Nurses:** Responsible for administering your chemotherapy treatments and answering your questions.

- **Radiation Oncologist:** Responsible for mapping out your radiation therapy.

- **Radiation Therapists:** The technicians who operate the machines and administer your therapy.

- **Registered Dietician:** A health professional with special training in diet and nutrition.

- **Reproductive Endocrinologist:** Specializes in the treatment of fertility issues for men and women.

- **Perinatologist or High-Risk Obstetrician:** Specializes in high-risk pregnancies.

- **Medical Geneticist:** Specializes in diagnostic and therapeutic procedures for patients with genetically linked diseases.

- **Psychologist, Psychiatrist, or Social Worker:** Professionals who can help you with your emotions before, during, and after your treatments.

Referrals can come from people you trust, such as your primary doctor, family, friends, or other breast cancer patients. Try and find a doctor who is part of a pre-treatment multidisciplinary conference. This is a group of doctors, which may include a surgeon, radiologist, and medical oncologist, who review and discuss your records and make recommendations regarding your particular cancer.

> I followed up on seeing my three doctors for three opinions on whether to have a mastectomy or a lumpectomy. The first doctor was much too old to give any current advice. I felt very discouraged by the second doctor's advice and had no empathy from this man--not a good sign. The third doctor listened to me for over an hour, to all the ins and outs I had been through. God bless him.
>
> —Bette H.

Appointments and Contacts

You will have a mind-boggling number of appointments. The *Appointments Worksheet* on page 28 and the *Contacts Worksheet* on page 23 will help you stay organized and remember who's who. Each specialist will probably assign you a new patient identification number. Record this ID number next to each contact. This enables your doctors, hospital billing, and insurance company to quickly access your records. It also helps to find a 24-hour pharmacy; you never know when you might need one. Since you will use these worksheets often, keep copies near your home phone for quick reference.

Doctors need to keep track of all of your prescriptions to make sure they work together. The same thing applies to your treatment team members. Make a copy of your *Contacts Worksheet* and share it with each specialist you see. This way everyone will stay in the loop and share important information when developing your treatment plan.

A word of caution: You can drive yourself crazy seeking too many opinions.

Choosing Your Treatment Team

Why spend time with someone you're not at ease with? It's important to be comfortable with your doctors and not be afraid to talk with them. Together you will decide your best treatment game plan. Take the time to figure out what you want and need from your team and what factors are going to be important to you during and after your care. The *Evaluate Your Doctor Worksheet* on page 30 will help you with this. Consider these factors when evaluating the facility your doctor is associated with:

- **Type of hospital:** Is it a designated cancer center or academic institution?

- **Type of accreditation:** Does the facility meet the highest standards?

- **Approach to care:** Do they treat breast cancer using multidisciplinary teams?

- **Location:** How close is the facility to you? Does it offer transportation?

- **Cost for services:** Is this facility covered by your health insurance?

- **Hospital privileges:** Does your treatment team have permission to use the hospital?

Opinions and Second Opinions

When making big decisions like buying a house or car, we usually shop around and investigate our options. This holds true for choosing your treatment team members. Just because you have seen one doctor doesn't mean you can't see another. You are entitled, and usually encouraged, to seek second opinions on all aspects of your treatment. Often, insurance companies require you to do so. Second opinions can give you confirmation and peace of mind, help you clarify information, and allow you to explore different doctors' personalities. Ask your primary care physician for names of several doctors who specialize in breast cancer. Check with your insurance company to see what it will pay for. Find out what records you will need and make sure each doctor receives them.

Sometimes you won't even know all your treatment options until you get another opinion. As you begin to learn about your options, call ahead and ask which ones that doctor provides. You are not limited to a certain treatment plan just because your doctor does not perform others.

Long-Distance Opinions

You may want to seek a second opinion from a medical facility or expert outside of your area. You can do this without even leaving your home. You will usually have to pay a fee for these services. The *Seeking a Second Opinion Worksheet* on page 32 will guide you. Below are a few of the facilities that provide a second opinion on your initial diagnosis and treatment options:

Cleveland Clinic
MyConsult Office H2-260
Cleveland Clinic
9500 Euclid Avenue
Cleveland, Ohio 44195

Phone:	800-223-2273 Ext.4322
	216-444-3223
Email:	eClevelandClinic@ccf.org
Website:	*http://eclevelandclinic.org/myconsult*

Johns Hopkins Medicine
Attn: Medical Second Opinion Team
5801 Smith Avenue, Suite 305
Baltimore, MD 21209-3611

Phone:	410-735-4339
Fax:	410-735-6670
Email:	medicalsecondopinion@jhmi.edu
Website:	*www.hopkinsmedicine.org/avon_foundation_breast_center/second_opinion.html*

Partners Online Specialty Consultations
Phone:	617-724-9295
	888-456-5003
Website:	*https://econsults.partners.org*

After a couple of consultations you will start to get a feel for your treatment options. Usually there is no rush, but you do not want to delay treatment and waste your time and energy by seeing too many specialists. Get as many opinions as you need to feel good.

Know Your Medical History

It's surprising and frankly a little annoying when you are asked to fill out similar forms again and again. Completing the *Medical History Worksheet* on page 34 will save you time and reduce the pressure of having to recall information at appointments.

Know Your Family History

Try as we might, we can't control our families. This applies to their medical history as well. Sometimes we are at a greater risk of certain diseases based on our family's history. Complete the *Family History Worksheet* on page 37 to help your doctor figure out your risk of certain diseases. Ask your family for help with this worksheet.

> **Never go to a doctor whose office plants have died.**
>
> —*Erma Bombeck*

Let Others Know

With whom you share your diagnosis and how much you choose to share is up to you. There will come a point when you will need to start letting certain people know. It helps to be prepared for a wide range of reactions and remember that cancer affects your family and friends as well.

Children react in varying ways depending on their ages, personalities, and developmental stages. If your children are in school, it helps to inform their teachers, principals, and school social workers of your situation. Cancercare.org suggests the following tips when speaking with children:

- Use simple language; do not overwhelm them with too much information.

- Tell them basic facts about breast cancer.

- Let them know that cancer is no one's fault and that they cannot "catch" your cancer.

- Encourage questions; reassure them that there are no dumb questions.

- Ask them what they would like to know.

- Accept their unwillingness to talk. Children will talk when they are ready.

The American Cancer Society provides easy-to-understand literature and support groups for all ages. Your doctors can also direct you to age-appropriate educational materials and resources. Keep talking to your children. Remember, they too are along on this journey, and like you, they are looking for reassurance and a sense of control.

The Waiting Game

Waiting to see a doctor or to get test results can be agonizing. This is the perfect time to address some paperwork and help take your mind off worrying. Did you get copies of your reports or lab results? Do you know when, where, and by whom you should be seen next? Tackling the following worksheets can give you a sense of control and keep you moving forward between each appointment.

Action Items

- Complete *Procedure Worksheets* as needed on pages 50-53.
- Record and file any *Medical Expenses* on pages 84-85.
- Record and file any *Insurance Claims* on pages 80-81.
- Record any new *Contacts* on pages 23-27.
- Record any new *Appointments* on page 28.

Contents

Patient Information

Name:	Phone:
Address:	Email:

Emergency Contact

Name:	Phone:
Address:	Email:

Emergency Contact

Name:	Phone:
Address:	Email:

Emergency Contact

Name:	Phone:
Address:	Email:

Primary Physician/Internist

Name:	Phone:	Fax:
Address:		Email:
Nurse:		Patient #:

Surgeon

Name:	Phone:	Fax:
Address:		Email:
Nurse:		Patient #:

Nurse Navigator

Name:	Phone:	Fax:
Address:		Email:

Contacts

Contacts

Medical Oncologist

Name:	Phone:	Fax:
Address:		Email:
Nurse:		Patient #:

Radiation Oncologist

Name:	Phone:	Fax:
Address:		Email:
Nurse:		Patient #:

Plastic Surgeon

Name:	Phone:	Fax:
Address:		Email:
Nurse:		Patient #:

Genetics Counselor

Name:	Phone:	Fax:
Address:		Email:

Anesthesiologist

Name:	Phone:	Fax:
Address:		Email:
Nurse:		Patient #:

OB/Gynecologist

Name:	Phone:	Fax:
Address:		Email:
Nurse:		Patient #:

Genetics Counselor

Name:	Phone:	Fax:
Address:		Email:

Contacts

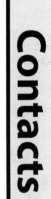

Hospital

Name:	Phone:	Fax:

Address:

Registration Phone Number:

Hospital Billing Contact:	Phone:

Insurance Carrier

Name:	Phone:	Fax:

Address:	Email:

Nurse:	Patient:

Disability Insurance Carrier

Name:	Phone:	Fax:

Address:	Email:

Nurse:	Patient:

Pharmacy

Name:	Phone:	Fax:

Address:

24-Hour Pharmacy

Name:	Phone:	Fax:

Address:

Nutritionist

Name:	Phone:	Fax:

Address:	Email:

Social Worker

Name:	Phone:	Fax:

Address:	Email:

Contacts

Therapist

Name:	Phone:	Fax:
Address:		Email:

Physical Therapist

Name:	Phone:	Fax:
Address:		Email:

Employer

Name:	Phone:	Fax:
Address:		Email:
Contact:		Phone:

Exercise Specialist

Name:	Phone:	Fax:
Address:		Email:

Legal

Name:	Phone:	Fax:
Address:		Email:

Certified Massage Therapist: Lymphatic Drainage

Name:	Phone:	Fax:
Address:		Email:

Support Group

Name:	Phone:	Fax:
Address:		Email:
Contact:		Phone:

Contacts

Contents

Family/Friends

Name:	Phone:
Address:	Email:

Name:	Phone:
Address:	Email:

Name:	Phone:
Address:	Email:

Name:	Phone:
Address:	Email:

Name:	Phone:
Address:	Email:

Name:	Phone:
Address:	Email:

Name:	Phone:
Address:	Email:

Name:	Phone:
Address:	Email:

Name:	Phone:
Address:	Email:

Name:	Phone:
Address:	Email:

Name:	Phone:
Address:	Email:

Appointments

You can keep track of new appointments using the worksheet below. Be sure to add any new contacts to your *Contacts Worksheet* as well. If your appointment involved some type of procedure you can record that information on the *Medical Procedures Worksheet*.

Date	Who you are seeing	Phone	Location	Purpose of Visit	Procedure

Appointments

You can keep track of new appointments using the worksheet below. Be sure to add any new contacts to your *Contacts Worksheet* as well. If your appointment involved some type of procedure you can record that information on the *Medical Procedures Worksheet*.

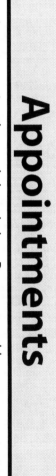

Date	Who you are seeing	Phone	Location	Purpose of Visit	Procedure

Evaluate Your Doctors

You can compare your visits and decide who you feel will make the best member of your treatment team. Place a check mark under each doctor's name if the factor applies to him or her. Choose which factors are most important to you when making your decisions.

Factor	Dr.:		Dr.:		Dr.:	
Easy to communicate with	☐ Yes	☐ No	☐ Yes	☐ No	☐ Yes	☐ No
Specializes in my type of cancer	☐ Yes	☐ No	☐ Yes	☐ No	☐ Yes	☐ No
Board Certified	☐ Yes	☐ No	☐ Yes	☐ No	☐ Yes	☐ No
Trustworthy/Good first impression	☐ Yes	☐ No	☐ Yes	☐ No	☐ Yes	☐ No
Explained my diagnosis clearly	☐ Yes	☐ No	☐ Yes	☐ No	☐ Yes	☐ No
Listened to me	☐ Yes	☐ No	☐ Yes	☐ No	☐ Yes	☐ No
Reacted well to my questions	☐ Yes	☐ No	☐ Yes	☐ No	☐ Yes	☐ No
Allowed visits to be recorded	☐ Yes	☐ No	☐ Yes	☐ No	☐ Yes	☐ No
Good body language	☐ Yes	☐ No	☐ Yes	☐ No	☐ Yes	☐ No
Easy to reach, returns calls quickly	☐ Yes	☐ No	☐ Yes	☐ No	☐ Yes	☐ No
Spent enough time with me	☐ Yes	☐ No	☐ Yes	☐ No	☐ Yes	☐ No
Has problem solving approach	☐ Yes	☐ No	☐ Yes	☐ No	☐ Yes	☐ No
Involved in new treatment studies	☐ Yes	☐ No	☐ Yes	☐ No	☐ Yes	☐ No
Clean, efficient office	☐ Yes	☐ No	☐ Yes	☐ No	☐ Yes	☐ No
Well-trained and helpful office staff	☐ Yes	☐ No	☐ Yes	☐ No	☐ Yes	☐ No
Convenient location	☐ Yes	☐ No	☐ Yes	☐ No	☐ Yes	☐ No
Hospital teaching affiliation	☐ Yes	☐ No	☐ Yes	☐ No	☐ Yes	☐ No
Good reputation	☐ Yes	☐ No	☐ Yes	☐ No	☐ Yes	☐ No
Payment plan	☐ Yes	☐ No	☐ Yes	☐ No	☐ Yes	☐ No
Mention complimentary therapies	☐ Yes	☐ No	☐ Yes	☐ No	☐ Yes	☐ No
Accounting department for Insurance & billing help	☐ Yes	☐ No	☐ Yes	☐ No	☐ Yes	☐ No
Total Check Marks:	___Yes	___ No	___Yes	___ No	___Yes	___ No

Evaluate Your Doctors

You can compare your visits and decide who you feel will make the best member of your treatment team. Place a check mark under each doctor's name if the factor applies to him or her. Choose which factors are most important to you when making your decisions.

Factor	Dr.:	Dr.:	Dr.:
Easy to communicate with	❑ Yes ❑ No	❑ Yes ❑ No	❑ Yes ❑ No
Specializes in my type of cancer	❑ Yes ❑ No	❑ Yes ❑ No	❑ Yes ❑ No
Board Certified	❑ Yes ❑ No	❑ Yes ❑ No	❑ Yes ❑ No
Trustworthy/Good first impression	❑ Yes ❑ No	❑ Yes ❑ No	❑ Yes ❑ No
Explained my diagnosis clearly	❑ Yes ❑ No	❑ Yes ❑ No	❑ Yes ❑ No
Listened to me	❑ Yes ❑ No	❑ Yes ❑ No	❑ Yes ❑ No
Reacted well to my questions	❑ Yes ❑ No	❑ Yes ❑ No	❑ Yes ❑ No
Allowed visits to be recorded	❑ Yes ❑ No	❑ Yes ❑ No	❑ Yes ❑ No
Good body language	❑ Yes ❑ No	❑ Yes ❑ No	❑ Yes ❑ No
Easy to reach, returns calls quickly	❑ Yes ❑ No	❑ Yes ❑ No	❑ Yes ❑ No
Spent enough time with me	❑ Yes ❑ No	❑ Yes ❑ No	❑ Yes ❑ No
Has problem solving approach	❑ Yes ❑ No	❑ Yes ❑ No	❑ Yes ❑ No
Involved in new treatment studies	❑ Yes ❑ No	❑ Yes ❑ No	❑ Yes ❑ No
Clean, efficient office	❑ Yes ❑ No	❑ Yes ❑ No	❑ Yes ❑ No
Well-trained and helpful office staff	❑ Yes ❑ No	❑ Yes ❑ No	❑ Yes ❑ No
Convenient location	❑ Yes ❑ No	❑ Yes ❑ No	❑ Yes ❑ No
Hospital teaching affiliation	❑ Yes ❑ No	❑ Yes ❑ No	❑ Yes ❑ No
Good reputation	❑ Yes ❑ No	❑ Yes ❑ No	❑ Yes ❑ No
Payment plan	❑ Yes ❑ No	❑ Yes ❑ No	❑ Yes ❑ No
Mention complimentary therapies	❑ Yes ❑ No	❑ Yes ❑ No	❑ Yes ❑ No
Accounting department for Insurance & billing help	❑ Yes ❑ No	❑ Yes ❑ No	❑ Yes ❑ No
Total Check Marks:	___ **Yes** ___ **No**	___ **Yes** ___ **No**	___ **Yes** ___ **No**

Seeking a Second Opinion

Type		Given By	
Address		Phone	
Email		Fax	
Records Needed		Date Sent	
Records Location			

After reviewing my records, do you agree with the first opinion? _____

_____

_____

_____

_____

_____

What are your recommendations? _____

_____

_____

_____

_____

_____

What are the advantages and risks of your options? _____

_____

_____

_____

_____

_____

Comments/Questions: _____

_____

_____

_____

_____

Seeking a Second Opinion

Type		Given By	
Address		Phone	
Email		Fax	
Records Needed		Date Sent	
Records Location			

After reviewing my records, do you agree with the first opinion? _____

_____

_____

_____

_____

_____

What are your recommendations? _____

_____

_____

_____

_____

_____

What are the advantages and risks of your options? _____

_____

_____

_____

_____

_____

Comments/Questions: _____

_____

_____

_____

_____

Medical History

The sections listed below are not meant to represent your entire medical history, just a brief summary. If you are uncomfortable writing anything down, leave the area blank or make a photocopy to fill in.

Personal History of Medical Problems (check all that apply)

- ☐ Alcoholism
- ☐ Alzheimer's
- ☐ Anxiety/Depression
- ☐ Arthritis
- ☐ Asthma
- ☐ Blood Disorders/Clots
- ☐ Bowel Disease
- ☐ Emphysema
- ☐ Gynecological problems
- ☐ Heart Disease
- ☐ Hepatitis

- ☐ High Blood Pressure
- ☐ High Cholesterol
- ☐ Hypoglycemia
- ☐ Kidney/Bladder problems
- ☐ Liver Disease
- ☐ Lung Disease
- ☐ Osteoporosis
- ☐ Stomach Problems
- ☐ Seizures
- ☐ Stroke

Family History of Cancer:
List any cancer your family members have had.

Family Member	Type of Cancer	Age at Diagnosis

Current Medications:
List all prescriptions, including over-the-counter medications, vitamins, and herbal medications.

Medicine	Dose	Times per Day	Why	For How Long

Medical History

Gynecological/Obstetric History

Date of last period ____/____/____

Age that you started menstruating: _____

Have you gone through menopause? ❑ Yes ❑ No If yes, at what age? _____

Do/did you use oral contraceptives? ❑ Yes ❑ No If yes, for how long? _____

Number of pregnancies, including miscarriages and abortions: _____

Number of births_____ Number of vaginal deliveries_____ Number of C-sections_____

Age at first full term pregnancy: _____

Have you had a hysterectomy? ❑ Yes ❑ No

If yes, were your ovaries removed? ❑ Yes ❑ No

Have you ever had an abnormal pap smear? ❑ Yes ❑ No If yes, when?_____

Is there a chance you could be pregnant? ❑ Yes ❑ No _____

Allergies or Reactions to Medicines/Food/Other Agents

Medication/Food/Item	Reaction or Side Effect

Surgical History

Operation	Date	Operation	Date

Medical History

Immunizations: Please list dates of last immunization.

Hepatitis A ____/____/____ Hepatitis B ____/____/____ Tetanus ____/____/____

Flu Shot ____/____/____ Pneumonia ____/____/____ Meningitis ____/____/____

Social History

Do you smoke? ☐ Yes ☐ No If yes, how many a day? ______ For how many years?______

Do you drink alcohol? ☐ Yes ☐ No If yes, how many drinks per week? ____________

Do you use recreational drugs? ☐ Yes ☐ No

If yes, which drugs? ________________________________

Do you have a religious preference? ☐ Yes ☐ No

If yes, please state: ________________________________

Marital status: ☐ Single ☐ Married ☐ Divorced ☐ Widowed

What type of work do you do? ________________________ ☐ Retired

Health Maintenance

Have you had a recent mammogram?	☐ Yes	☐ No	Date: __________
Have you had a recent pap test?	☐ Yes	☐ No	Date: __________
Have you had a recent colonoscopy?	☐ Yes	☐ No	Date: __________
Have you had a recent bone density scan?	☐ Yes	☐ No	Date: __________
Have you had a recent dental exam?	☐ Yes	☐ No	Date: __________
Do you have regular physicals?	☐ Yes	☐ No	Date: __________
Do you examine your breasts regularly?	☐ Yes	☐ No	Date: __________

Notes: ________________________________

Family History

Your family medical history should include at least three generations. Gather information about your grandparents, parents, uncles, aunts, siblings, and children.

Are you Jewish?　　　　　❑ Yes　❑ No

Are you African American?　❑ Yes　❑ No

What region or country did your father's ancestors come from?_____

What region or country did your mother's ancestors come from? _____

Family Relation	Current Age	Age at Death	Cancer Type	Age at First Cancer Diagnosis	Additional Health Issues	Age at Second Cancer Diagnosis
Your Mother's Family						
Mother						
Maternal Grandfather						
Maternal Grandmother						
❑ Aunt　❑ Uncle						
❑ Aunt　❑ Uncle						
❑ Cousin						
❑ Cousin						
❑ Niece　❑ Nephew						
Your Father's Family						
Father						
Paternal Grandfather						
Paternal Grandmother						
❑ Aunt　❑ Uncle						
❑ Aunt　❑ Uncle						
❑ Cousin						
❑ Cousin						
❑ Niece　❑ Nephew						
Your Siblings						
❑ Sister　❑ Brother						
❑ Sister　❑ Brother						
❑ Sister　❑ Brother						
❑ Sister　❑ Brother						
Your Children						
❑ Daughter　❑ Son						
❑ Daughter　❑ Son						
❑ Daughter　❑ Son						
❑ Daughter　❑ Son						

Medications

Record all prescriptions and over-the-counter medicines. Be sure to inform your doctors regarding any changes in prescriptions, known allergies, or side effects that you might experience.

Pharmacy: _____

Phone: _____

Fax: _____

Medication Name	Refill Number	Ordered By	Dose	Start Date	End Date	What is it For?	Directions	Side Effects

Medications

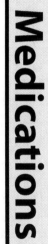

Record all prescriptions and over-the-counter medicines. Be sure to inform your doctors regarding any changes in prescriptions, known allergies, or side effects that you might experience.

Pharmacy: _____   Phone: _____   Fax: _____

Medication Name	Refill Number	Ordered By	Dose	Start Date	End Date	What is it For?	Directions	Side Effects

Document Storage

Type of Document	Contacts/Representatives	Storage Location
Accounting & Taxes	Name:	
	Phone:	
Bank Accounts	Name:	
	Phone:	
Business Documents	Name:	
	Phone:	
Car Insurance	Name:	
	Phone:	
Car Loans	Name:	
	Phone:	
Car Titles	Name:	
	Phone:	
Credit Cards	Name:	
	Phone:	
Death Certificate	Name:	
	Phone:	
Disability Insurance	Name:	
	Phone:	
Divorce Certificates/ Decrees	Name:	
	Phone:	
Driver's License	Name:	
	Phone:	
Durable Power of Attorney	Name:	
	Phone:	
Estate Planning	Name:	
	Phone:	
Financial Planning	Name:	
	Phone:	
Green Cards	Name:	
	Phone:	
Guardians	Name:	
	Phone:	
Home Insurance Policy	Name:	
	Phone:	

Document Storage

Type of Document	Contacts/Representatives		Storage Location
Health Insurance Policy	Name:		
	Phone:		
Inheritances & Gifts	Name:		
	Phone:		
IRAs	Name:		
	Phone:		
Investments	Name:		
	Phone:		
Life Insurance Policy	Name:		
	Phone:		
Living Will & Will	Name:		
	Phone:		
Marriage Certificates	Name:		
	Phone:		
Mortgages	Name:		
	Phone:		
Organ Donation	Name:		
	Phone:		
Passport	Name:		
	Phone:		
Personal Effects	Name:		
	Phone:		
Property Titles	Name:		
	Phone:		
Retirement Account	Name:		
	Phone:		
Stocks & Bonds	Name:		
	Phone:		
Social Security Card	Name:		
	Phone:		
Trusts	Name:		
	Phone:		
Work Information	Name:		
	Phone:		

Notes

> *To be prepared is half the battle.*
>
> *- Miguel Cervantes*

chapter 2

Know What You're Facing

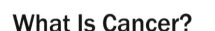

What Is Cancer?

You hear the term "cancer" or "the big C" all the time and you know it's not a good thing, but what exactly is it? Cancer is the general name for a group of more than 100 diseases in which cells in a certain part of the body begin to grow and divide out of control. Cells normally grow and divide to produce new ones in a controlled and orderly manner. However, sometimes new cells continue to grow and divide when they are not needed. These uncontrolled groups of cells can form a tumor. Not all tumors are cancerous. A benign tumor is not dangerous to your health, whereas a malignant tumor has the potential to be very dangerous if left untreated.

Ask your treatment team for guidance in gathering information pertaining to your cancer, helping you maximize your valuable time. Slowing down to make well-informed, rational decisions will allow you to maintain a sense of control over your emotional and physical recovery.

What Is Breast Cancer?

Cancers come in all shapes and sizes, and breast cancer is no exception. Breast cancer refers to a cancer that has started in the breast. There are approximately fifteen types of breast cancer, each requiring its own course of treatment. The type of breast cancer you have will depend on many factors, like where your tumor is located and whether it has spread to other sites in your body. When learning about your breast cancer, it helps to have a basic understanding of the anatomy of the breast. Normal breast structures include the following: *(See Figure 2.1)*

- **Nipple:** Area where milk leaves the breast

- **Areola:** Dark area surrounding the nipple

- **Lobules:** Glands that produce milk

- **Ducts:** Tiny tubes that bring the milk from the lobules out to the nipple

- **Stroma:** Connective tissue and supporting cells that surround the ducts & lobules

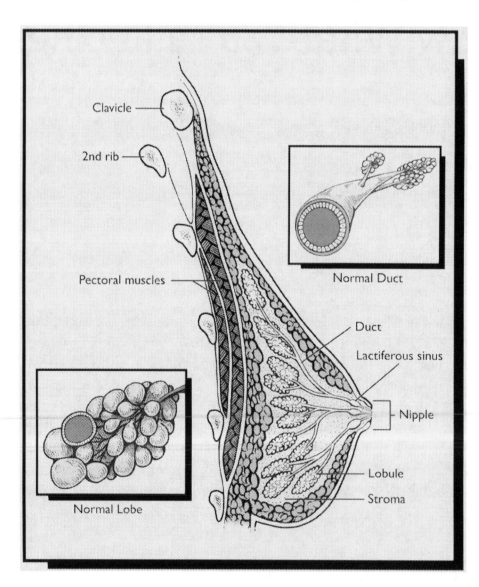

Figure 2.1

Breast cancers can sometimes spread through the **lymphatic system,** which plays an important role in the body's defenses and in its immune system. **Lymph nodes,** which are a part of this system, are glands that act as filters to stop bacteria and cellular waste from entering the blood stream. They are connected by **lymph vessels,** which carry lymph fluid away from the breast. Sometimes breast cancer cells can enter lymphatic vessels and begin to grow in lymph nodes.

Most of the lymphatic fluid leaving the breast is drained through the lymph nodes under the armpit (called axillary nodes). Fluid can also be drained by nodes in other areas, such as inside the chest (internal mammary nodes) and either above the collarbone (supraclavicular nodes) or below it (infraclavicular nodes). *(See Figure 2.2)*

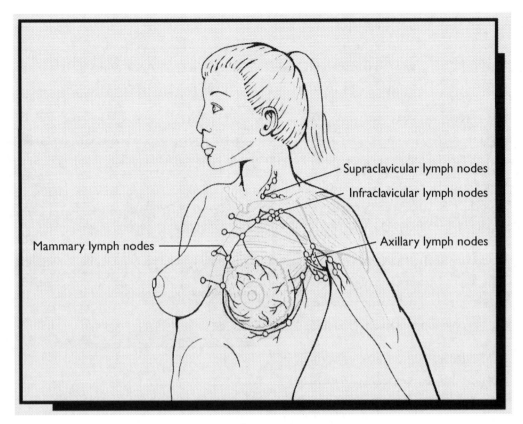

Figure 2.2

Types of Breast Cancer

Cancers are sometimes named for where they start. Most breast cancers begin in the cells that line the ducts and are referred to as ductal cancers. Others can begin in the cells that line the lobules and are called lobular cancers. When cancer cells are confined to the organ in which they started, this is referred to as **in situ cancer.** Cancer cells that spread beyond the layers of cells where the cancer started and into nearby tissue are called **invasive cancer cells** or **infiltrating cancer.** *(See Figure 2.3)*

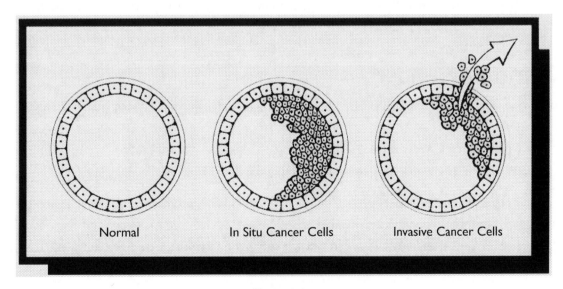

Figure 2.3

These more common types include:

- **Ductal Carcinoma in Situ (DCIS):** DCIS refers to cancer cells in the lining of the milk duct that have not invaded the surrounding breast tissue. (*See Figure 2.4*)

- **Invasive Ductal Carcinoma (IDC):** Cancer cells form in the lining of the milk duct, break free from the duct wall and invade the surrounding breast tissue. (*See Figure 2.4*)

- **Invasive Lobular Carcinoma (ILC):** ILC starts in the milk-producing lobule and invades the surrounding breast tissue.

- **Metastatic:** Metastatic cancer is cancer that has spread from the primary site (the place where it started) to other places in the body.

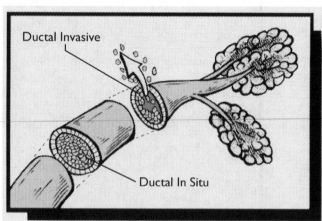

Figure 2.4

- **HER-2/neu-Positive Breast Cancer:** An aggressive form of breast cancer caused by too much of a gene called HER2 in tumor cells. Women with breast cancer whose tumors test positive for HER2 overexpression may be candidates for trastuzumab or lapatinib.

- **Hormone Receptor-Positive:** This refers to breast cancer cells that have receptors (proteins) that bind to the hormones estrogen and/or progesterone and depend on estrogen or progesterone to grow. Antiestrogen therapies, such as tamoxifen or aromatase inhibitors, work effectively against this type of cancer cell.

Less-Common Cancers

A small number of cancers start in other tissues. These include but are not limited to:

- **Medullary Carcinoma:** A rare form of invasive ductal cancer with cells that resemble the color of brain tissue (the medulla).

- **Triple Negative:** A type of breast cancer in which cancer cells lack estrogen and progesterone receptors. In addition they do not have an excess of the HER2/neu protein on their surfaces. Hormone therapies are not effective against this type of cancer, nor are drugs that target HER-2/neu.

- **Tubular Carcinoma:** Invasive cancer with cells that look like little tubes.

- **Inflammatory Breast Cancer (IBC):** IBC is caused by cancer cells in the lymph vessels of the skin that make the skin red and block the drainage of fluid from the skin.

- **Paget's Disease:** Cancer that starts in the ducts and then moves to the nipples.

- **Adenocystic Carcinoma:** Named for their microscopic appearance, the cancer cells in this condition resemble adenoid (glandular) and cystic cells.

- **Phylloides tumor:** A tumor that develops in the connective tissue of the breast.

- **Carcinosarcoma:** A malignant tumor that is a mixture of carcinoma (cancer of epithelial tissue, which is skin and tissue that lines or covers the internal organs) and sarcoma (cancer of connective tissue, such as bone, cartilage, and fat).

- **Unknown Primary Cancer:** Cancer that has spread to a lymph node in the armpit without an obvious primary tumor.

- **Apocrine breast cancer:** Cancer found in the apocrine gland, which is responsible for secreting fat droplets into breast milk.

Who Is at Risk for Breast Cancer?

We don't think of men as vulnerable to breast cancer, but they can get it too. Certain risk factors make some people more likely than others to develop breast cancer. These risk factors include:

For Both Women and Men:
- Age: Your chances of getting breast cancer increase as you age.

- Obesity

- Personal history of a previous breast cancer

- Family history of breast cancer

- Genetic risk factors: Carrying the BRCA1 or BRCA2 gene

- Previous radiation therapy to the chest

- Dense breasts

- Lack of physical activity

- Drinking alcohol

For Women:
- Being overweight or obese after menopause

- Early menstrual onset (before age 12)

- Menopause

- Race (breast cancer is diagnosed more often in Caucasian women)

For Men:

- High estrogen levels

- Klinefelter syndrome: A condition in which men have more than one X chromosome

- Use of finasteride (a drug used to treat and prevent prostate cancer)

- Liver disease

- Certain testicular conditions (undescended testicle, surgical removal of one or both testicles)

Additional Diagnostic Testing

Like patients with other conditions, breast cancer patients undergo more than one test to confirm the diagnosis and determine the extent of the cancer. These tests might include:

- **Biopsy:** This is the surgical removal of a small piece of tissue or tumor to examine the cells. Biopsies are performed in the following ways:

    - Core needle
    - Fine needle
    - Guided ultrasound
    - Stereotactic needle
    - Excisional
    - Incisional
    - Vacuum-assisted

- **3D Mammography:** Also known as tomosynthesis. A type of mammogram that produces a 3D image of the breast and gives doctors a clearer view through the overlapping structures of breast tissue.

- **Blood Counts:** Blood is drawn and examined to evaluate red and white blood cells, platelets, electrolytes, and hemoglobin, among other factors.

- **Bone Scan:** This procedure involves injecting a small amount of a radioactive substance into the bloodstream in order to see if cancer has spread to the bones.

- **Computed Tomography (CT or CAT) Scan:** A specialized x-ray that can detect small tumors and metastasis.

- **Mammogram:** An x-ray of the breast.

- **Magnetic Resonance Imaging (MRI):** This test uses powerful magnetic fields to image the breast.

- **Positron Emission Tomography (PET) Scan:** This procedure involves injecting a small amount of radioactive glucose (sugar) into the bloodstream and then using a scanner to see if the cancer has spread to other areas of the body.

- **Ultrasound:** This is the use of high-frequency sound waves to help determine if a lump is solid or filled with fluids.

The *Diagnostic Procedure Checklist* on page 50 will help you keep track of the tests you have. The *Medical Procedures Worksheet* on page 51 allows you to keep track of who performed the procedure and where it was performed.

Genetic Testing

Do you have your father's dimple or your mother's piercing blue eyes? You share common gene traits with your relatives, some of which have been passed down from generation to generation. Sometimes (not very often) a breast cancer gene can run in families. If you or your doctors suspect this to be the case, you might want to proceed with genetic testing. Genetic testing analyzes your DNA (Deoxyribonucleic acid; the control center of every cell) to look for mutations that indicate you are at a higher risk for developing a specific disease or disorder. A simple but expensive blood test can be done to check for these mutations. BRCA1 and BRCA2 are two genes that are thought to be connected to breast cancer.

If you decide to pursue genetic tests, check with your insurance provider for coverage and make an appointment with a certified genetics counselor. Use the *Questions for the Genetic Counselor* on page 53 when discussing your testing options.

Diagnostic Procedure Checklist

Diagnostic Procedure Checklist

Procedure	Date	Copy of My Results	Completed Procedure Worksheet?
❑ Mammogram		❑ Yes ❑ No	❑ Yes ❑ No
❑ Ultrasound		❑ Yes ❑ No	❑ Yes ❑ No
❑ Lumpectomy		❑ Yes ❑ No	❑ Yes ❑ No
❑ Core Needle Biopsy		❑ Yes ❑ No	❑ Yes ❑ No
❑ Fine Needle Aspiration		❑ Yes ❑ No	❑ Yes ❑ No
❑ Clips		❑ Yes ❑ No	❑ Yes ❑ No
❑ Sterotactic Biopsy		❑ Yes ❑ No	❑ Yes ❑ No
❑ Surgical Biopsy		❑ Yes ❑ No	❑ Yes ❑ No
❑ Mammotome Biopsy		❑ Yes ❑ No	❑ Yes ❑ No
❑ MRI		❑ Yes ❑ No	❑ Yes ❑ No
❑ CT Scan		❑ Yes ❑ No	❑ Yes ❑ No
❑ PET Scan		❑ Yes ❑ No	❑ Yes ❑ No
❑ Bone Scan		❑ Yes ❑ No	❑ Yes ❑ No
❑ Lumpectomy		❑ Yes ❑ No	❑ Yes ❑ No
❑ Mastectomy		❑ Yes ❑ No	❑ Yes ❑ No
❑ Other:		❑ Yes ❑ No	❑ Yes ❑ No
❑ Other:		❑ Yes ❑ No	❑ Yes ❑ No
❑ Other:		❑ Yes ❑ No	❑ Yes ❑ No
❑ Other:		❑ Yes ❑ No	❑ Yes ❑ No
❑ Other:		❑ Yes ❑ No	❑ Yes ❑ No
❑ Other:		❑ Yes ❑ No	❑ Yes ❑ No
❑ Other:		❑ Yes ❑ No	❑ Yes ❑ No

Medical Procedures

Use this worksheet to track your procedures and assist you in keeping your records organized.

Type of procedure:_____ Date:_____/_____/_____

Who performed it? _____

What were my results?_____

Who interpreted the results? _____

Where are my tissue samples being stored? _____

How long will tissue samples be stored? _____

How do I get a physical copy of my results? _____

Where are my records being kept? _____

❑ Discharge Summary   Location:_____

❑ Pathology Reports   Location:_____

❑ Imaging Reports (Before and After Surgery)   Location:_____

❑ Copies of Films (X-Ray, CT, MRI, Bone Scans) Location:_____

❑ Other   Location:_____

❑ Specimen   Location:_____

Payment Method:

Insurance Claim #: _____ Date:_____/_____/_____

Out of Pocket: Check #:_____   ❑ Cash   ❑ Credit Card

Follow-Up & Notes _____

_____

_____

_____

_____

_____

Medical Procedures

Medical Procedures

Use this worksheet to track your procedures and assist you in keeping your records organized.

Type of procedure:_____ Date:_____/_____/_____

Who performed it? _____

What were my results?_____

Who interpreted the results? _____

Where are my tissue samples being stored?_____

How long will tissue samples be stored? _____

How do I get a physical copy of my results? _____

Where are my records being kept? _____

❑ Discharge Summary   Location:_____

❑ Pathology Reports   Location:_____

❑ Imaging Reports (Before and After Surgery)   Location:_____

❑ Copies of Films (X-Ray, CT, MRI, Bone Scans)   Location:_____

❑ Other   Location:_____

❑ Specimen   Location:_____

Payment Method:

Insurance Claim #: _____ Date:_____/_____/_____

Out of Pocket: Check #:_____   ❑ Cash   ❑ Credit Card

Follow-Up & Notes _____

_____

_____

_____

_____

_____

Medical Procedures (vertical side text)

Questions for the Genetic Counselor

Why do you feel I am a candidate for genetic testing?_____
_____

What are the implications of genetic test results for me and my family?_____
_____

What other genes can be tested for besides BRCA1&2?_____
_____

Are some people better candidates than others in a family? _____
_____

Is genetic discrimination something I need to be concerned about?   ❑ Yes   ❑ No

Will insurance cover testing for me and my family?   ❑ Yes   ❑ No

If not, are there financial assistance programs to help cover the costs?   ❑ Yes   ❑ No

Should I share my results with my healthcare professionals?   ❑ Yes   ❑ No

Are there any support networks for individuals who are found to have a hereditary breast cancer syndrome?_____
_____

What if I do not want to do genetic testing? _____
_____

What about my family's options? _____
_____

Where can I get more information?_____
_____

What is the best way to communicate with you? _____
_____

Additional questions/comments: _____
_____
_____
_____
_____

Notes

chapter

3

Understanding Your Pathology Report

Reading Your Report

You don't have to have a medical degree to be successfully treated for breast cancer. However, in order to help form your plan of attack, you do need to know what type of breast cancer you have. Your pathology report tells you about your type of cancer. Your doctors are going to base their treatment advice on the results of this report. You want a breast pathologist to have written your report. If one did not, ask your doctor about obtaining your slides and where you can send them for a second opinion by a breast pathologist.

You do not need to understand every single aspect of your pathology report. When using the *Pathology Worksheet* on page 64, ask as many or as few questions as you feel comfortable with.

What's on the Report?

Type of Breast Cancer

The pathology report will tell you whether the cancer is non-invasive or invasive. The cancer will most likely be named based on its location.

Tumor Size and Location

The size of your tumor is measured in centimeters and will be noted on your report. *(See Figure 3.1)*

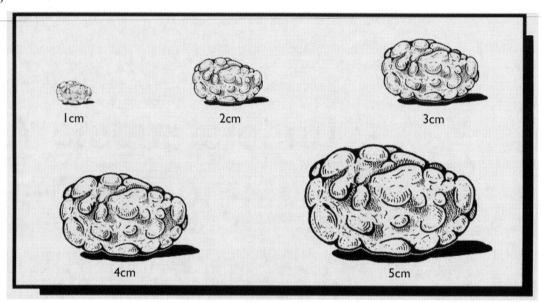

Figure 3.1

Tumors can also be classified by their location. The breast is divided in to five areas: upper right quadrant, upper left quadrant, lower right quadrant, lower left quadrant, and central (the nipple area). Tumor locations may be described as if on the face of a clock (for example, "upper right quadrant at 1 o'clock"). Your report may also tell you whether additional cancer was found in the same quadrant (multifocal) or if it was found in additional quadrants (multicentric). *(See Figures 3.2 and 3.3)*

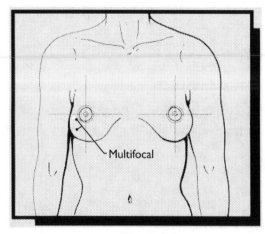

Figure 3.2

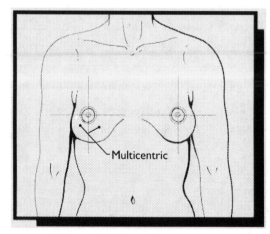

Figure 3.3

Margins

Margins refer to the area of tissue surrounding a tumor when it is removed. The tumor and the surrounding tissue are rolled in a special ink so that the outer edges, or margins, are clearly visible under a microscope. A pathologist checks the tissue to see if any cancer remains on the outer edges. Clean margins, also known as negative margins, mean a lower risk of recurrence. A positive margin can result in another surgery to ensure clean margins. Sometimes remaining cancer cells are close to the edge of the tissue, but not exactly at the edge. If this is the case, the surgeon may recommend additional surgery. *(See Figure 3.4)*

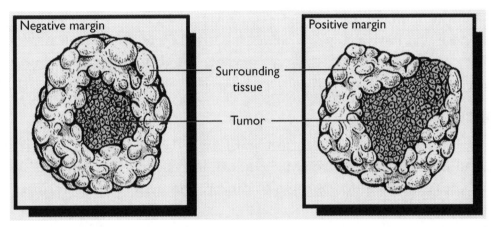

Figure 3.4

Lymphatic Involvement

Surgery is often performed to remove and dissect your lymph nodes to determine whether the cancer has spread (metastasized) from the breast area to the nodes. If it has, there is a higher chance that the cancer cells have also entered into the bloodstream and spread to other sites in your body. This is important to know because it will affect your treatment plan.

The tumor is also examined by the pathologist to see if the cancer has invaded the surrounding blood or lymphatic vessels. They may also count the number of vessels associated with the tumor. High numbers of vessels, or a known invasion, are suggestive of a rapidly growing, aggressive tumor. The number of involved lymph nodes and vessels will be stated on your report.

Nuclear Grade and Cell Differentiation

The pathologist will evaluate the size and shape of the nucleus inside the tumor cells and the percentage of cells that are in the process of dividing. He or she will then assign a grade. A low-nuclear-grade cancer tends to grow more slowly than a high-nuclear-grade cancer.

Cell differentiation refers to how much the tumor cells resemble the original (normal) cell. Tumor cells are examined microscopically to determine the degree of change from normal and are then graded or classified as:

- **Well-Differentiated Cells (Low Grade, Grade 1)**
  These cells look very similar to normal cells. This type of cancer tends to be slow growing.

- **Moderately Differentiated Cells (Intermediate Grade, Grade 2)**
  These cells have changed but still resemble the parent cell.
  This type of cancer grows faster than grade 1 but slower than grade 3.

- **Poorly Differentiated Cells (High Grade, Grade 3)**
  These cells have lost most of the characteristics of normal cells.
  This type of cancer tends to be fast growing.

- **Undifferentiated Cells (High Grade, Grade 4)**
  These cells have changed dramatically from their original cell and have an abnormal appearance. This type of cancer tends to be fast growing.

Breast Cancer Stages

Cancer staging is a system that is used to identify whether your cancer has spread from its original site, and if so, how far. The TNM classification system is the standard system used by the medical field to identify different types of cancer. This system looks at three factors when determining the stage of your cancer: the size of the tumor (T), whether lymph nodes are involved (N) or (pN), and whether the cancer has metastasized, or spread beyond the breast to other areas of the body (M). Your tumor, nodes, and metastasis are first given a score as shown in Table 3.1.

Table 3.1: TNM SCORES
Tumor Size:
TX: A primary tumor cannot be found
T0: There is no evidence of primary tumor
Tis: Carcinoma In situ (DCIS, LCIS or Paget's Disease)
T1: Tumor is between 0 and 2 cm
T2: Tumor is between 2-5 cm
T3: Tumor >5 cm
T4: Tumor that has grown into chest wall or skin
Node Status:
N0: No lymph nodes are involved   **N2:** 4-9 lymph nodes are involved
N1: 1-3 lymph nodes are involved   **N3:** 10 or more lymph nodes are involved
Metastasis:
MX: Cannot find any distant spread of cancer
M0: There is no distant spread
M1: There is a spread to distant organs present

[American Joint Committee on Cancer (AJCC) TNM system]

Once your scores have been assigned for each component, they are combined to determine the stage of your cancer as shown in Table 3.2. (*See Figures 3.5, 3.6, 3.7, 3.8, 3.9*)

Table 3.2: TNM STAGING			
Stage	**Tumor Size**	**Lymph Node Involvement**	**Metastasis (Has it spread?)**
Stage 0	**Tis:** any size	**N0:** Negative	**M0:** None
Stage 1A	**T1:** <2 cm	**N0:** Negative	**M0:** None
Stage 2A	**T0:** no cancer found in breast	**N1:** Positive	**M0:** None
	T1: <2 cm	**N1:** Positive	**M0:** None
	T2: 2-5 cm	**N0:** Negative	**M0:** None
Stage 2B	**T2:** 2-5 cm	**N1:** Positive	**M0:** None
	T3: <5 cm	**N0:** Negative	**M0:** None
Stage 3A	**T0:** no cancer found in breast	**N2:** Positive	**M0:** None
	T1: <2 cm	**N2:** Positive	**M0:** None
	T2: 2-5 cm	**N2:** Positive	**M0:** None
	T3: <5 cm	**N1:** Positive	**M0:** None
	T3: <5 cm	**N2:** Positive	**M0:** None
Stage 3B	**T4:** any size with chest wall or skin involvement	**N0, N1, N2** or **N3:** Positive or Negative	**M0:** None
Stage 3C	**Any size**	**N3:** Positive:	**M0:** None
Stage 4	**Any size**	**N0, N1, N2** or **N3:** Positive or Negative	**M1:**Yes

[American Joint Committee on Cancer (AJCC) TNM system]

Figure 3.5

Stage 0

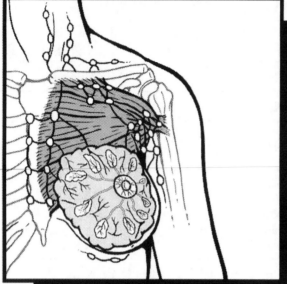

T = Any size N = Negative M = None

Figure 3.6

Stage 1

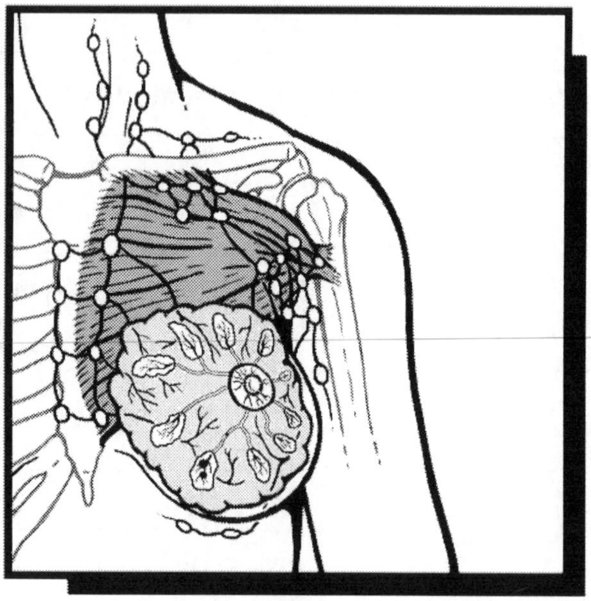

T = < 2cm N = Negative M = None

Figure 3.7

Stage 2

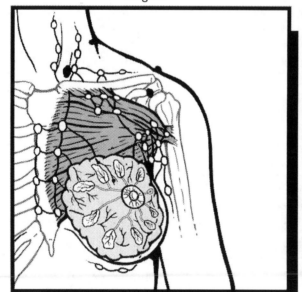

Any of these:

T = No cancer found N = Positive M = None

T = < 2cm   N = 1-3 Positive M = None
T = 2-5cm N = Negative   M = None
T = 2-5cm N = 1-3 Positive M = None
T = > 5cm N = Negative   M = None

Figure 3.8

Stage 3

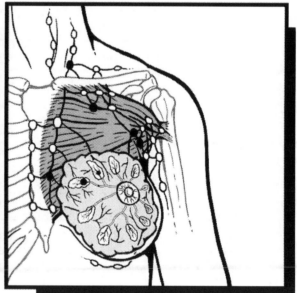

Any of these:

T = No cancer found N = 4-9 Positive M = None

T = < 2cm   N = 4-9 Positive M = None
T = 2-5cm N = 4-9 Positive M = None
T = > 5cm N = 1-3 positive M = None
T = any size N = 1-9 positive M = None
T = any size N = 10+ Positive M = None

Figure 3.9

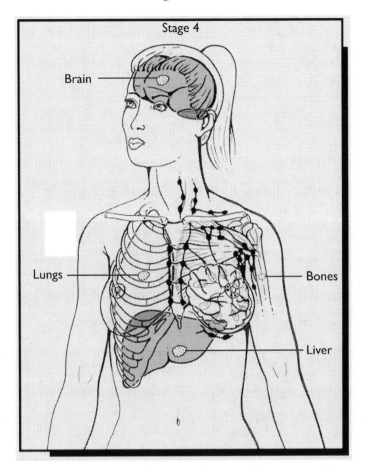

Tumor Markers

Tumor markers are hormones, proteins, or parts of proteins that are made by a tumor or by the body in response to a tumor. These markers are substances that show up in the blood, urine, or tumor. Your pathology report may include information on the following:

- **Hormone Receptors:** Hormone receptors are molecules on the surface of cells. These receptors recognize hormones circulating in the blood stream. Both estrogen (ER) and progesterone (PR) hormones influence breast maturation and can sometimes promote the development of breast cancer. Cancer cells can become stimulated to grow when estrogen binds with the cancer cell hormone receptors.

  ER-positive and PR-positive cells are cancer cells that have these receptors.

  ER-negative or PR-negative cells are cancer cells without these receptors.

- **HER-2/neu oncongene:** Human epidermal growth factor receptor-2 gene (HER-2/neu) is the gene that is responsible for making HER-2 proteins. Cancers that have too many of these proteins tend to be more aggressive. This can occur by the HER-2/neu gene making too many copies of itself (gene amplification) or when there are too many receptors (over-expression) of the HER-2/neu gene.

HER-2/neu positive are cancer cells that produce the oncongene.

HER-2/neu negative are cancer cells that don't produce the oncongene.

- A tumor that is ER negative, PR negative, and HER-2/neu negative is referred to as a **triple negative tumor.**

Understanding Risk

As you gather treatment information, your doctors will talk to you about reducing the risk of your breast cancer returning. It is important to know whether they are referring to your relative risk or your absolute risk.

- **Relative risk** is used to compare risks between two groups. It is the number that tells you how different treatments, such as radiation therapy, can change your risk as compared to not having radiation therapy.

- **Absolute risk** is the size of your own risk. Absolute risk reduction is the number of percentage points by which your own risk changes if you do something, like having radiation therapy. The size of your absolute risk reduction depends on what your risk is to begin with.

Let's say that after having a successful lumpectomy, your surgeon tells you that your risk of cancer returning in the same breast is about 30%. However, if you choose to have radiation therapy after your lumpectomy, you can reduce this risk of the cancer coming back by 60%. This is the **relative risk** decrease. Your **absolute risk** of the cancer coming back then drops from 30% to 10%.

Knowing the difference between relative risk and absolute risk could profoundly affect your treatment decisions. Make sure your doctors explain risks in terms of absolutes and how each treatment affects your type of cancer. Ask as many questions as necessary to understand the advantages and disadvantages of all of your treatment options.

> The time is now to receive all the love people want to give you. When I opened up to receiving that love, I gained so much confidence and insight that I got to see a much more meaningful me.
> The love filled me up and helped give me strength to be who I truly am.
>
> —Sue B.

Fertility Issues

Sadly, women do get breast cancer while pregnant or before they have had the opportunity to have children. The good news is that breast cancer does respond well to treatment during pregnancy. The bad news is that some types of treatment cause a permanent loss of fertility. Your doctors will look at many factors when determining which treatments are best for you. The *Pregnancy Questions* on page 66 and the *Fertility Questions* on page 67 will guide you as you discuss your treatment options. Regardless of the treatment path you choose, it is wise to also seek professional emotional support at this time.

Clinical Trials

Clinical trials are research programs designed to evaluate new methods of treating cancer. Clinical trials are carefully considered treatment plans that show great promise. They look for options that may prove to be more effective than the current standard treatments, with fewer side effects and lower rates of recurrence. If your doctors feel you are a candidate for a trial, the *Clinical Trial Questions* on page 68 can help guide you through the process.

> The best advice I could give to a person diagnosed with breast cancer is to stay positive. Every day, scientists are making new discoveries and breakthroughs in the fight against breast cancer. Never, ever just surf the Internet looking for information or statistics [or a] prognosis.
>
> The Internet can be a very scary place with incorrect, outdated, and very broad information. Remember, you are an individual; you are a statistic of one.
>
> —Judy H.

Pathology Worksheet

Your report may or may not contain all of the information below. Some of the information will not be available to you until after surgery.

What type of biopsy did I have? _____

Who wrote my pathology report?_____

      Address: _____

      Phone: _____

      Email: _____

Are they a breast cancer specialist?   ❑ Yes   ❑ No

If no, is second opinion recommended?   ❑ Yes   ❑ No

Do I have a copy of the report?   ❑ Yes   ❑ No

Where are my samples being kept? _____

      Address: _____

      Phone: _____

      Email: _____

What is the tissue size?   Greatest Dimensions _____cm

                      Additional Dimensions _____cm x _____cm

How long are tissue samples being kept? _____

How can I obtain my samples? _____

What type of cancer do I have?_____

Cancer Stage: ❑ 0   ❑ I   ❑ 2A   ❑ 2B   ❑ 3A   ❑ 3B   ❑ 3C   ❑ 4

Are my margins clean?   ❑ Negative/Clean   ❑ Positive/Involved

Hormone receptor status:

    ❑ ER positive (+)/PR positive (+)   ❑ ER negative (-)/PR positive (-)

    ❑ ER positive (+)/PR negative (-)   ❑ ER negative (-)/PR (-)

HER-2/neu status:

    ❑ Positive

        ❑ By IHC: Tests for over-expression of the HER2 protein

        ❑ By FISH: Tests for too many copies of the actual gene

    ❑ Negative

    ❑ Triple Negative: ER negative/PR negative (-)/HER-2neu negative (-)

Pathology Worksheet

What is the size of my tumor? _____

Cell differentiation grade: ❑ 1 ❑ 2 ❑ 3 ❑ 4

Cell's architectural pattern: _____

Position: _____ O'clock ❑ Multifocal ❑ Multicentric

Tumor Site:

❑ Right Side ❑ Left Side ❑ Central (Nipple)

❑ Upper Inner Quadrant ❑ Lower Inner Quadrant

❑ Upper Outer Quadrant ❑ Lower Outer Quadrant

Was there necrosis? ❑ Not identified ❑ Present, focal ❑ Present, central

Was there blood vessel or lymphatic vessel invasion? ❑ Yes ❑ No

Tumor grade: ❑ 1 ❑ 2 ❑ 3

How were my lymph nodes examined _____

Were my lymph nodes involved? ❑ Yes ❑ No

Number of Nodes Removed: _____ Number of Nodes Negative: _____

Number of Nodes that are Involved (Tested Positive):

❑ N0: No lymph nodes involved ❑ N2: 4-9 lymph nodes involved

❑ N1: 1-3 lymph nodes involved ❑ N3: 10 or more lymph nodes involved

Am I at an increased risk for lymphedema? ❑ Yes ❑ No

Who should I see next? _____

What are my treatment options? _____

What is my prognosis? _____

Where can I get more information? _____

Additional comments/questions: _____

_____

_____

Pregnancy Questions

I am pregnant. What are my treatment options? _____

_____

_____

If I continue my pregnancy, how will it affect my treatment outcomes? _____

_____

_____

How will treatments affect my baby? _____

_____

_____

Can I delay treatments until after my delivery?   ❏ Yes   ❏ No

Will I be able to breast feed?   ❏ Yes   ❏ No

How soon after treatments end can I get pregnant? _____

Can you refer me to a High Risk Obstetrician? _____

Where can I get more information? _____

What is the best way to communicate with you? _____

Additional questions/comments: _____

_____

_____

_____

_____

_____

_____

_____

_____

_____

_____

_____

_____

Pregnancy Questions

Fertility Questions

Will I continue to have menstrual periods? ❑ Yes ❑ No

If not, will they return? _____

Should I use birth control? ❑ Yes ❑ No

If yes, what type? _____

How will treatments (surgery, radiation, chemo, hormonal) impact my fertility? _____

_____

_____

_____

_____

Are there drugs I can use with less potential for infertility? _____

_____

If I want to pursue embryo freezing, is there time to do so without it impacting my survival

outcome? ❑ Yes ❑ No

How long after treatments will it take for my period to return? _____

_____

What should I use for contraceptives? _____

_____

If my fertility returns, how long should I wait before becoming pregnant? _____

_____

Will treatments affect my sex life? _____

_____

Can I have children after my cancer? ❑ Yes ❑ No

Will my future children be at risk based on my treatment choices? _____

_____

Where can I get more information? _____

_____

Can you refer me to a fertility specialist? _____

_____

What is the best way to communicate with you? _____

_____

Additional questions/comments: _____

_____

_____

Clinical Trial Questions

Why do you think I am a good candidate for a trial?_____

_____

What results can reasonably be expected in my case?_____

_____

Who is sponsoring this trial and what are they trying to learn from this study? _____

_____

What phase is the trial in?

❑ **Phase 1:** This phase evaluates how the drug should be given, how often, and the dose that is most effective while causing the least side effects. Initially, a small number of participants are enrolled.

❑ **Phase 2:** Treatments or drugs continue to be tested for their safety and effectiveness. They usually focus on a particular type of cancer.

❑ **Phase 3:** The new treatment is compared to the best current standard treatment. Large numbers of participants are enrolled. You may be randomly assigned to either the new treatment group or standard treatment group.

❑ **Phase 4:** After the new treatment or drug has been approved it goes through a surveillance phase. During this phase more information is gathered about its side effects, risks, and who would benefit the most from its use.

What are the currently accepted standard treatments, and how do they compare?_____

_____

What is involved in terms of tests, treatments, and additional time commitments? _____

_____

Will I have to travel? ❑ Yes ❑ No If yes, where? _____

Will I be hospitalized during the treatment? ❑ Yes ❑ No If so, how long:_____

What are the possible short-term risks? _____

_____

_____

What are the possible long-term risks? _____

_____

_____

Clinical Trial Questions

How will this study affect my daily living? _____
_____

What safety measures are built in to the trial? _____
_____

What will my follow-up care be? _____
_____

What are the financial commitments associated with a trial? _____
_____

Will my insurance provider cover this?   ❑ Yes   ❑ No

How long will the trial last and what if I want to stop? _____
_____

What are the results of the trial so far? _____
_____

Who is in charge of my care during the study? _____

Can I speak with other participants?   ❑ Yes   ❑ No

Who is in charge of my care after the study? _____

How will I know if the treatment worked? _____
_____

Where can I get more information? _____

What is the best way to communicate with you? _____

Additional questions/comments: _____
_____
_____
_____
_____
_____
_____

Notes

*A good companion shortens
the longest road.*

- Turkish Proverb

chapter 4

Embracing Support Systems

You Don't Have to Go It Alone

Battles are won by the coordinated efforts of troops working toward a common goal. Millions of people have successfully survived breast cancer using the same tactics. Many individuals and groups are waiting to help you win your fight against breast cancer. Take advantage of them, starting with the people you know.

Your friends and family want to help you. They are your biggest fans who want to cheer you on. They too are looking for a sense of control and can feel frustrated that they aren't able to do more. Allowing them to help you helps them in return. There will be times when you will want and need help. How much you need will depend on your treatment. You might need a ride to an appointment, some help around the house, or a just a friend to talk to.

Sometimes our family and friends make excellent capable companions and caregivers. Sometimes they don't. How do you decide who should do what? It depends. A capable companion is someone who can be relied on to be a second set of eyes and ears; accompanying you to appointments, recording information at doctor visits, and providing emotional support during treatment. A caregiver is someone helping you in some way—physically, emotionally, spiritually, or financially.

Think about who is best suited to help you. Many times your capable companion is someone other than your caregiver. Although they mean well, loved ones are not always the best choice to be capable companions since they are often as distressed as you are.

Help for Your Helpers

Sometimes we get so caught up in what's happening to us that we forget about those who are trying to help. Caregiving can be both rewarding and stressful. Caregiver.org suggests you share the following guidelines with your caregivers to help them help you.

> When you accept a role as a capable companion and a caregiver you need to understand that your "reality" will be altered and that you need to take care of your physical and emotional needs as well as your loved one's. You need to be all that you can be to assist your loved one through this journey.
>
> So take your own inventory often and seek assistance as needed.
>
> Communication is critical and can be difficult. It is important that you know when to speak, when to listen, and when to express love and support. This is not as easy as it sounds, because the view from the passenger seat is different.
>
> —Kirk B.

- **Acknowledge your emotions.** Recognize that the cancer diagnosis has a tremendous impact on you as well. Do not hold in your emotions.

- **Talk about your feelings.** Often caregivers feel overwhelmed by the increased responsibilities that a loved one's diagnosis brings. One of the best ways to cope with your fears, stress, and uncertainties is to join a support group. Or confide in a trusted friend.

- **Take care of yourself first.** No, you are not being selfish. Keep in mind that while you are taking on new responsibilities, you are still allowed a life of your own.

- **Gather information.** The more you understand about the cancer diagnosis, the better prepared you are to help your loved one.

- **Communicate.** Different issues will arise in each phase of treatment. Talk about how you are both feeling and ask exactly how you can help.

- **Recognize a "new normal."** Acknowledge that your home life, daily activities, and social life will change for a period of time.

- **Accept help.** You can't know and do everything, nor should you. Let others perform tasks that they are willing and able to do.

- **Take breaks.** Avoid burnout by keeping your life balanced.

- **Know your limits.** Come to terms with feeling overwhelmed, acknowledge your limits, and be firm when deciding what you can and cannot handle on your own.

People with goals succeed because they know where they're going.

- Earl Nightingale

chapter

Staying on Track

Addressing Your Practical Matters

Cancer changes your world but doesn't stop it. You will still need to pay bills, maintain work and school schedules, and take care of daily chores and activities. The trick is learning how to manage it all while seeking treatment. It helps to assemble a "practical matters" team. Your team members might include a financial planner or accountant, a health insurance representative, a lawyer, an estate planner, your friends, and your family. The sooner you start organizing your practical matters, the sooner you can focus your energy on your treatment and healing.

Balance Your Budget

There is no way around it: cancer is expensive. Even with excellent insurance coverage, your medical expenses can add up. The best way to prepare for the financial realities of a cancer diagnosis is to tackle one aspect at a time, starting with balancing your budget. Understanding your financial situation can help you gain a sense of control and guide you as you make decisions.

Continuing to Work

If you are currently working, the amount of time you'll need to take off will depend on your treatment plan, your financial situation, and your emotional and physical state. Ask your doctors to estimate how many days off you will need to help you plan. Remember, how much information you want to share with your employer is up to you. You cannot be discriminated against because of your illness. Two laws are in place to specifically protect you:

- **Family and Medical Leave Act (FMLA):** This law requires businesses with more than fifty employees to allow you up to twelve weeks of unpaid leave in order to take care of yourself or a sick family member.

- **Americans with Disabilities Act (ADA):** This law protects employees from being discriminated against because of illness. Breast cancer is considered a disability for the purpose of this law.

If you feel you are being discriminated against, keep records. Write down whom you spoke with, what was said, and what response you received. This information can be useful if you need to take further action.

Navigating the Insurance Maze

Have you ever found out after the fact that a standard medical procedure isn't covered by your insurance policy? It's not surprising that the same thing can happen during your cancer treatments. That's why, before making any treatment decisions, it's important you fully understand your health insurance policy by taking some time and reading through it. Use the *Insurance Questions* on page 78 when meeting with an insurance representative to answer all your questions. Learn what will and won't be covered, what deductibles are in place, and what protocols must be followed—in language you understand. Once you have a clear understanding of your policy, you can make informed treatment decisions and understand the financial implications of your choices.

> **A hospital bed is a parked taxi with the meter running.**
>
> —*Groucho Marx*

Insurance Paperwork

You've probably had an issue with a phone bill or cable bill when you spoke to a different person each time you called the company and had to explain the situation over and over. This can also happen with insurance companies. Lessen the chances of this by asking your insurance provider to assign you a case manager. You will then speak with the same person every time. Another way to stay organized is to create a filing and record-keeping system for insurance-related paperwork such as claims, benefits, and doctor's letters.

It is helpful if you can get in the habit of:

- Filling in the *Insurance Claims Tracker* on page 80.

- Making copies of all bills and filing them with your insurance company immediately. (Many medical providers will do this for you. Make sure you know if yours has so that you do not file duplicate claims.)

- Filling in the *Insurance Correspondence Worksheet* on page 82 each time you speak with an insurance representative.

Keep apples with apples, oranges with oranges. In other words, keep similar documents together for record-keeping purposes. You might want to wait to pay your bills until you receive your estimate of benefits (EOB) statement for each fee. This will help you keep track of your out-of-pocket expenses and deductibles, and avoid billing errors.

What to Do If You Are Uninsured

Not everyone has health insurance. If you don't, you do have some options. Find out if you qualify for:

- **Aid to Families with Dependent Children (AFDC):** This government program provides assistance to low-income families with children under the age of 18.

- **Health Risk Insurance Pools:** Health insurance risk pools are special programs created by state legislatures to provide a safety net for the "medically uninsurable" population. These are people who have been denied health insurance coverage because of pre-existing health conditions or who can only access private coverage that is restricted or has extremely high rates.

- **Hospital Assistance:** Ask a social worker or caseworker at the facility where you will be seeking treatment to help you find financial assistance. Inquire about:
  - Drug assistance programs run by pharmaceutical companies
  - Generic drug options
  - Hospital payment plans
  - Clinical trials

- **Medicaid:** This program provides medical assistance for individuals with low income. Each state has varying qualifications. Check with the hospital social worker to find out if you're eligible.

- **Medicare:** Program that provides health insurance to retired people who:
  - Are U.S. citizens sixty-five years old or older who worked for ten years in Medicare-covered employment
  - Have received Social Security disability payments for two years
  - Are permanently disabled

- **Social Security:** You may qualify for assistance if you meet the requirements to be considered disabled by the U.S. Social Security Administration.

- **Veterans Affairs:** The U.S. Department of Veterans Affairs provides health benefits to veterans and their dependents.

Managing Bills

It's easy to start feeling overwhelmed when all the bills start arriving. Talk to your doctors about your financial concerns using the *Financial Questions* on 83. To stay on top of bills and reduce stress:

- Create a record-keeping system for medical-related expenses.

- Complete the *Medications Worksheet* on page 38.

- Complete the *Medical Expenses Worksheet* available on page 84.

> *Taking care of your practical matters really frees you up, allowing you to spend your time and energy elsewhere. In fact, the very act of taking care of them and checking them off of your "to-do list" will make you feel better instantly. As you move forward on your journey, keep the path clear by addressing issues as they arise and seeking help when needed.*
>
> —Cara N.

Make Your Wishes Known

Learning you have cancer highlights the importance of making your wishes known. A practical matter that many people put off—cancer patients and non-cancer patients alike—is creating legal documents. Whether or not you are sick, the following documents can help eliminate "second guessing" by family members and doctors:

- **Advance directives,** sometimes called **living wills,** are instructions given by you that specify what actions should be taken for your health in the event you are no longer able to make those decisions due to illness or incapacity. They inform the medical team of what levels of care you do or do not want, including withholding certain treatments, such as life support.

- **Medical power of attorney,** sometimes called a **durable power of attorney,** is a document that allows you to appoint someone else to make decisions about your medical care if you are no longer able to. Choosing a power of attorney can be an emotional task. Discuss the responsibilities of this position with whomever you are considering before assigning this important role.

- **Estate planning** is the process of arranging your financial affairs so that your belongings will be distributed according to your wishes after your death. Often these are designed to help avoid undue taxation.

- **A legal guardian,** sometimes called a **ward,** is a person who has the legal authority (and the corresponding duty) to care for your personal and property interests.

Let someone on your practical matters team assist you with balancing your budget, organizing your insurance, and creating your legal documents. Remember, you are not alone. Family and friends are looking for ways to help you.

Insurance Questions

What is my yearly deductible and co-pay? _____

When is it applied? _____

What treatments are covered by my policy? _____

_____

_____

What procedures or visits require pre-authorization? _____

_____

_____

Are all of my hospitalization costs covered?   ❑ Yes   ❑ No

If not, what isn't covered? _____

_____

_____

What will I have to pay for? _____

_____

_____

Up to what amount? _____

Do I have a maximum limit? _____

Does my coverage travel with me if I go out of state?   ❑ Yes   ❑ No

Are my doctor visits covered? _____

Can I choose a doctor out of network?   ❑ Yes   ❑ No

If yes, what are my costs? _____

_____

Is reconstructive surgery covered?   ❑ Yes   ❑ No

Do I have to have reconstruction immediately or can I wait?   ❑ Yes   ❑ No

Is breast prosthesis covered?   ❑ Yes   ❑ No

Are my prescriptions covered?   ❑ Yes   ❑ No

Are necessary over-the-counter items covered?   ❑ Yes   ❑ No

Insurance Questions

Are second opinions covered?   ❑ Yes   ❑ No

Are emergency room visits covered?   ❑ Yes   ❑ No

Does my policy cover a clinical trial?   ❑ Yes   ❑ No

Am I covered if I have a recurrence?   ❑ Yes   ❑ No

Am I eligible for additional coverage?   ❑ Yes   ❑ No

Can I be assigned a case manager?   ❑ Yes   ❑ No

If yes, who? _____

What can I do if a claim is denied? _____

_____

Additional questions/comments: _____

_____

_____

_____

_____

_____

_____

_____

_____

_____

_____

_____

_____

_____

Insurance Questions

Insurance Claims Tracker

Insurance Claims Tracker

Record all insurance claims as you receive them. Use the last column "year to date" total to keep track of how much you have paid out-of-pocket for the year and towards your annual deductible. Use this information for tax purposes.

Insurance Carrier: _____ Policy Number: _____

Billing Address: _____ Phone: _____

Case Manager: _____ Phone: _____ Email: _____

Claim #	Date of Service	Service Provided	Date of Payment	Amount Billed	Amount Covered	Amount Not Covered	Amount Paid by You	Year-to-Date Deductible

Insurance Claims Tracker

Record all insurance claims as you receive them. Use the last column "year to date" total to keep track of how much you have paid out-of-pocket for the year and towards your annual deductible. Use this information for tax purposes.

Insurance Carrier: _____ Policy Number: _____ Phone: _____

Billing Address: _____

Case Manager: _____ Phone: _____ Email: _____

Claim #	Date of Service	Service Provided	Date of Payment	Amount Billed	Amount Covered	Amount Not Covered	Amount Paid by You	Year-to-Date Deductible

Insurance Correspondence

Keep track of every correspondence with your insurance company by filling out the worksheet below.

Claim Number	Date	Time	Name of Contact	Call Reference Number
Written Correspondence sent to:		Issue Discussed:		Outcome:

Claim Number	Date	Time	Name of Contact	Call Reference Number
Written Correspondence sent to:		Issue Discussed:		Outcome:

Claim Number	Date	Time	Name of Contact	Call Reference Number
Written Correspondence sent to:		Issue Discussed:		Outcome:

Financial Questions

Who in your office handles billing questions?

Name: _____ Phone: _____ Email: _____

Who in your office handles insurance issues?

Name: _____ Phone: _____ Email: _____

Do you offer payment plans? ❏ Yes ❏ No

Explain: _____

_____

Do you offer or know of any prescription assistance programs? ❏ Yes ❏ No

Explain: _____

_____

Are there generic drugs that I can use? ❏ Yes ❏ No

Explain: _____

_____

Do you know of any programs to help cover my treatment costs? ❏ Yes ❏ No

Explain: _____

_____

Do you offer free or reduced rates for parking or transportation to and from treatments?

❏ Yes ❏ No

Explain: _____

_____

Where can I find free or reduced rate lodging? _____

Where can I find free or reduced counseling for myself? _____

Who offers free or reduced counseling for my family? _____

Is there somewhere I can get a free wig or other personal items? _____

_____

Additional questions/comments: _____

_____

Medical Expenses

Medical Expenses

Having accurate records of all of your medical expenses will help you save money in tax returns, insurance reimbursements, and insurance annual caps. Create a folder to keep track of all of your receipts for any items related to your medical care. These categories may include but are not limited to:

- Travel expenses
- Mileage
- Insurance premiums
- Co-payments
- Prescription drugs
- Medical supplies

- Physical therapy
- Complementary therapy
- Doctor's office visits
- Eye glasses & contacts
- Hearing aids
- Prosthesis

- Dental expenses
- Counseling & therapy
- Preventive check-ups
- Wigs
- Compression sleeve
- Home health care

Date	Expense Category	Method of Payment	Receipt	Amount You Paid	Total
			☐ Yes ☐ No		
			☐ Yes ☐ No		
			☐ Yes ☐ No		
			☐ Yes ☐ No		
			☐ Yes ☐ No		
			☐ Yes ☐ No		
			☐ Yes ☐ No		
			☐ Yes ☐ No		
			☐ Yes ☐ No		
			☐ Yes ☐ No		
			☐ Yes ☐ No		
			☐ Yes ☐ No		
			☐ Yes ☐ No		

Medical Expenses

Having accurate records of all of your medical expenses will help you save money in tax returns, insurance reimbursements, and insurance annual caps. Create a folder to keep track of all of your receipts for any items related to your medical care. These categories may include but are not limited to:

- Travel expenses
- Mileage
- Insurance premiums
- Co-payments
- Prescription drugs
- Medical supplies

- Physical therapy
- Complementary therapy
- Doctor's office visits
- Eye glasses & contacts
- Hearing aids
- Prosthesis

- Dental expenses
- Counseling & therapy
- Preventive check-ups
- Wigs
- Compression sleeve
- Home health care

Date	Expense Category	Method of Payment	Receipt		Amount You Paid	Total
			☐ Yes	☐ No		
			☐ Yes	☐ No		
			☐ Yes	☐ No		
			☐ Yes	☐ No		
			☐ Yes	☐ No		
			☐ Yes	☐ No		
			☐ Yes	☐ No		
			☐ Yes	☐ No		
			☐ Yes	☐ No		
			☐ Yes	☐ No		
			☐ Yes	☐ No		
			☐ Yes	☐ No		
			☐ Yes	☐ No		

Notes

Part II
Treatment Information

Several different therapies are available to help you treat your breast cancer. This section breaks down a variety of those options. Together, you and your doctors will determine which ones are best for you. Each chapter provides a brief overview and worksheets to help you succeed in navigating that particular treatment goal.

- **Chapter 6** reviews lymph node and breast surgery options.

- **Chapter 7** addresses post-mastectomy options.

- **Chapter 8** reviews radiation treatments.

- **Chapter 9** explores hormonal and targeted therapy options.

- **Chapter 10** introduces you to the language and concepts of chemotherapy.

- **Chapter 11** examines nutrition therapy.

- **Chapter 12** discusses the benefits of exercise.

- **Chapter 13** introduces you to complementary therapies.

- **Chapter 14** talks about what you might encounter in your aftercare.

- **Chapter 15** addresses the issue of recurrence.

Worksheets Quick Reference Guide

> *Believe you can and you're halfway there.*
>
> *- Theodore Roosevelt*

chapter 6

Surgical Strategies

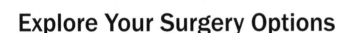

Explore Your Surgery Options

The main goals of surgery are to get rid of the cancer and keep it from coming back. There are two different types of initial surgeries: lymph node surgery to examine your nodes and breast surgery to remove the tumor. They can both take place during the same operation, or not. The *Questions for the Surgeon* on page 97 can help provide a starting point for making your decisions along with the *Surgical Treatment Options Worksheet* on page 99.

Lymph Node Surgery

Your lymph nodes will be examined before or during your breast surgery to determine if your cancer has spread into your lymph node area. Your lymph nodes are divided into three levels in the breast. Your surgery may involve removing nodes from one level or from several. This is done by either an axillary node dissection or a sentinel node biopsy.

- **Axillary node dissection** is a procedure that usually involves removing nodes from levels I and II in the armpit region. When all levels of nodes are removed the procedure is called a complete axillary dissection. A pathologist will examine the removed tissue to determine whether or not the cancer has spread and to what extent. The term negative nodes means there was no cancer found in your lymph nodes. If cancer is found, the nodes are called positive. The number of positive nodes found, if any, will help determine your treatment choices.

- **Sentinel node biopsy** is a procedure that involves the removal and examination of the first nodes (sentinel) to which the cancer cells are likely to have spread from the primary tumor. The sentinel nodes act as the gatekeepers to the rest of the lymphatic nodes. They identify the lymphatic chain and nodes most likely to indicate whether the cancer has metastasized (spread) to the regional lymph node area. Your surgeon can locate the sentinel nodes by injecting blue dye, radioactive particles or a combination of both into your breast. The first nodes to turn blue or radioactive are the sentinel nodes. If the sentinel nodes are cancer-free, the other nodes are likely to be cancer-free as well. Your surgeon will discuss your further options if your sentinel nodes are positive.

Breast-Conserving Surgery

One surgical option is breast-conserving surgery, which removes the tumor and varying degrees of the remaining breast tissue. There are two types of breast-conserving surgeries. They differ based on the size of the incision (cut) and how much breast tissue needs to be removed.

- **Lumpectomy:** The surgeon removes the tumor and a small portion of surrounding tissue. The skin is not removed unless the tumor is adhering to it. This surgery is sometimes called a tylectomy when a wider area of tissue surrounding the tumor needs to be removed. *(See Figure 6.1)*

- **Partial, Segmental Mastectomy or Quadrantectomy:** The surgeon removes the tumor along with a larger area of tissue around the tumor and possibly the overlying skin. A portion of the lining of the chest wall muscle and skin might also be removed. *(See Figure 6.2)*

Mastectomy Surgery

Another surgical option is some type of mastectomy, which removes the breast as well as the tumor. These surgeries include:

- **Total or simple mastectomy:** The surgeon removes all of the breast tissue, the nipple, and areola. The pectoral muscle, however, is not involved. Sometimes the lymph nodes under the arm are also removed.

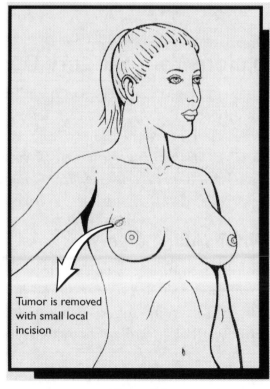

Tumor is removed with small local incision

Figure 6.1

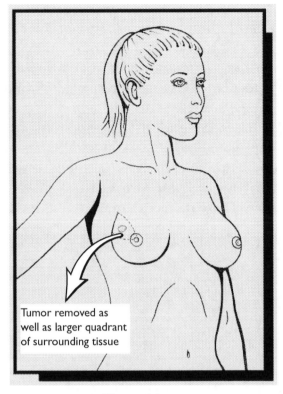

Tumor removed as well as larger quadrant of surrounding tissue

Figure 6.2

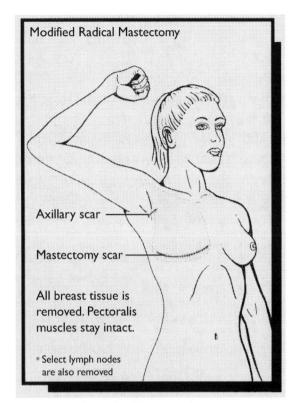

Modified Radical Mastectomy

Axillary scar

Mastectomy scar

All breast tissue is removed. Pectoralis muscles stay intact.

* Select lymph nodes are also removed

Figure 6.3

- **Modified radical mastectomy:** The surgeon removes all of the breast tissue, the nipple, areola, the lining of the pectoral muscle, and the axillary (underarm) lymph nodes. *(See Figure 6.3)*

- **Skin-sparing mastectomy:** The surgeon removes the breast tissue around the areola, nipple, and possibly lymph nodes. The excess skin and covering of the pectoral muscle is saved (spared) and used in the reconstruction of the breast. This type of surgery can be performed with either a modified radical or simple mastectomy.

- **Prophylactic mastectomy:** The surgeon performs a simple mastectomy before cancer has been found. Patients with an extremely high risk of developing breast cancer can choose to have a prophylactic (preventive) mastectomy to reduce their risk of getting breast cancer.

- **Nipple-sparing mastectomy:** The surgeon performs a mastectomy in which the breast tissue is removed but the skin and nipple areolar complex are preserved. This technique is ideal for patients with small peripheral tumors or those high-risk patients considering prophylactic mastectomy.

Ask your surgeon to draw or show you pictures of what the surgery will remove as well as what you will look like afterward. If you are also considering reconstructive surgery make sure you talk to your surgical oncologist before making decisions. The type of breast surgery you choose will influence your reconstructive choices.

Pre-Operative Planning

We've all been guilty of worrying—it's natural and part of human nature. But not worrying is easier said than done. Anything you can do to minimize stress can only work in your favor—realizing what you have control over can help reduce anxiety. You can't control the surgery but you can control what you know. Getting the answers to all of your questions ahead of time will lower stress and pre-op anxieties. The *Pre-Operative Questions* on page 101 will help you get ready, both mentally and physically. It's perfectly acceptable to schedule additional appointments with your doctor before surgery, enabling you to prepare for your recovery.

Travel light. You don't want to be burdened with having to carry a lot of things, especially after your surgery. Pack only what you will need for your hospital stay. Leave your valuable items such as jewelry, money, and credit cards at home. These items can make things easier for you:

- Loose-fitting front-opening clothing

- Slip-on shoes

- Surgeon-recommended bra

- Toothpaste and toothbrush

- Cell phone

- Reading material

Get your home ready for when you return. It helps to make your space as user-friendly as possible for after surgery. Keep items you will use often by your bedside or where you will be recuperating, especially if you have drains or have elected to have abdominal surgery. It can be helpful to:

- Purchase a camisole top with drain bulb pockets

- Fill your prescriptions ahead of time

- Keep a phone and list of important contacts near you

- Keep a TV remote and reading materials on nightstand

- Set up your caregiver's schedule

- Designate one person to communicate all your news

Day of Surgery

Some things never change. If you've ever checked into a hospital, you know the drill. Once you arrive at the hospital you will need to check in and fill out consent forms which explain the procedure you will undergo, including any emergency procedures. If you think you will be too nervous or unable to focus, ask for your consent forms to be mailed to you ahead of time. This will also let you be prepared if you have questions about them.

An anesthesiologist (the doctor who "puts you under") will most likely meet with you before surgery and will want to know every type of substance you are putting in your body, and that means everything. This is not the time to worry if you eat poorly, drink too much, or use recreational drugs. The anesthesiologist needs to be prepared for any and all possible reactions you might have during the surgery. It is extremely important to be frank with your anesthesiologist—your life can literally depend on it.

Post Surgery

Coming out of surgery and off drugs is probably not the best time to receive post-operative instructions. It's highly advised that your capable companion is present when talking with your doctors about your home care. The *Surgery Follow-Up Questions* on page 106 will help with taking notes. Remember to ask for a copy of your surgery information and record it on the *Treatment Summary Worksheet* on page 177.

Side Effects

Most surgeries come with side effects. Be sure to ask which ones you should look out for and who you should talk to about them. Keep track of any reactions on the *Side Effects Worksheet* on page 104. Below are some common post-operative issues.

Drain Bulbs

Drain bulbs are used to collect fluids that can build up after surgery. They are inserted by attaching a tube with a plastic bulb at the end to your tissue after a mastectomy, reconstructive surgery or an axillary dissection. The length of time bulbs are in place will vary from person to person. Before going home, make sure you have clear instructions on how to care for your bulbs, how to record your fluids, and what to look for. The *Drain Bulb Questions* & *Drain Bulb Care Worksheets* on pages 102-103 will help ensure you get the answers you need.

Seromas

Incision lines sometimes develop a buildup of fluid at the surgical site called a **seroma.** This is the most common side effect after surgery. Your surgeon may need to remove the fluid with a small needle to alleviate any further fluid buildup and pain, while monitoring the site for infection.

Numbness

Incision lines can have a decreased sensitivity at the surgical site. It often takes up to a year to see what feeling comes back and how much numbness will be residual. Over time you will become more aware of your post-surgical anatomy and what areas provide sensation and those that do not.

Tugging, Tightness, and Pain

It's common after surgery to experience tightness or a pulling sensation near your incisions. This will lessen over time. If movement becomes too restricted, you run the risk of developing a rare condition called **frozen shoulder,** which can occur due to scarring. Speak with your surgeon regarding appropriate exercises to regain your full range of motion.

Lymphedema

Lymphedema is painful swelling in the hand or arm of the surgical side due to lymph fluid build-up, and can sometimes occur with the removal and/or radiation treatment of axillary lymph nodes. Lymphedma occurs between 2% and 3% of the time following a sentinel node biopsy and between 15% and 20% of the time after an axillary dissection. Signs to look for include:

- Swelling, pain, or redness in the arm

- Feeling of tightness, heaviness, or fullness in the arm

- Feeling of tightness in the skin or a thickening of the skin

- Tight fit of rings, watches, or bracelets

The American Cancer Society recommends taking the following precautions to lessen your chances of developing lymphedema:

- Treat infections of the affected arm and hand right away.

- Wear gloves when doing house or garden work.

- Keep skin clean and well-moisturized.

- Use the unaffected arm when having blood drawn, getting injections, or having blood pressure taken.

- Avoid sunburn and excess heat from saunas, hot baths, tanning, and other sources.

- Do not cut nail cuticles.

- Avoid carrying heavy items on the surgical arm side.

- Use an electric razor when shaving anywhere.

- Use insect repellant when outdoors.

- Avoid injuries, including scratches and bruises, to the at-risk arm.

Ask your surgeon to write a prescription for a compression sleeve, which is an elasticized garment that is custom-fitted to your arm, and helps with pain and swelling caused by lymphedema.

Emotional Impact

There are few things more nerve-wracking than waiting for test results. Often the emotional side effects of surgery last longer and have a greater impact than the physical ones, and it can take time to adapt to your new appearance. Navigating intimate relationships can also take an emotional toll. It helps to know that your emotions often are all over the place and eventually, they really will settle down.

A "New" You

Yes, you are going to look different; you just had surgery. How different you look will depend on many factors, including your surgical choices. It is perfectly normal if you're hesitant to look at the "new" you after any surgery. Some people want to do it immediately, others want to wait. You might want to be alone when you look at your body or have someone with you for emotional support. Remember, your appearance will change as time passes and you heal.

A significant part of your post-treatment care is monitoring your breast(s) frequently. If you find yourself having difficulty accepting your new appearance, seek support from other breast cancer patients as well as your doctors. You can also switch your focus on other aspects of your appearance that are within your control. Go ahead; buy that new lipstick color or pair of shoes you've been eyeing.

Intimacy Issues

Just because you had cancer doesn't mean you can't be intimate. In fact, it brings many couples closer together. Still, all sorts of thoughts might be racing through your head. How will I look? How will my partner react? What do I tell someone new? Will I ever feel sexy? It is very possible you will experience changes in your sex drive due to emotional and physical issues. Each treatment choice can impact your desire for sex for a variety of reasons. Learning ahead of time what to expect can help ease the transition back to intimacy. Talking openly and honestly with your partner and treatment team will help you with your intimate relationships.

> Resuming intimacy can be tricky. It was for me. First, there was the problem of a sore surgical site. Next, I had to figure out how to deal with the razor stubble on my head rubbing on the sheets. Then we had to navigate around my sensitive skin from radiation.
>
> Just when I thought it was safe, my libido plummeted from chemo-induced menopause and sex became painful. Fortunately I was able to talk with my doctors and remedy the situation. A good sense of humor and a patient, loving partner go a long way.
>
> —Cara N.

Navigating Depression

Having cancer stinks. Acknowledging this can go a long way in helping you manage your emotions. It's perfectly natural to experience feelings of sadness and loss and even the occasional period of depression. You have been through a lot. However, if feelings of depression linger or become more severe it is important to seek help. Recognizing the signs of depression is the first step. These can include but are not limited to:

- A chronic sense of hopelessness
- Uncontrolled crying spells
- Insomnia or inability to get out of bed
- Lack of interest in everything
- Obsessing about your health
- Loss of appetite and energy
- Suicidal thoughts

Seeking help is the second step in treating depression. If you are experiencing prolonged signs of depression do not hesitate to speak with your treatment team—or anyone for that matter. Counseling and medications have proven to be extremely beneficial in treating depression.

Post-Surgery Exercises

Sometimes you don't know what you've got till it's gone. Boy, is that true of your arm mobility after surgery. It's going to be important to regain your arm and shoulder range of motion. This can help decrease side effects and allow you to return to your normal daily activities. Talk with your doctor before starting any exercises. Some exercises are appropriate soon after surgery; others need to wait until drains are removed. Ask which exercises would be good for you and when you can start doing them. Stop exercising and speak with your doctor if you start experiencing:

- Pain or swelling
- Heaviness in your arm
- Nausea, headaches, or visual disturbances

Brushing your hair, your teeth, your dog—they're all good arm exercises as well. Whenever possible, use your surgical arm for eating, grooming and other normal movements, but remember, don't overdo it.

Questions for the Surgeon

Are you board certified?   ❏ Yes   ❏ No

Are you a part of a cancer treatment team?   ❏ Yes   ❏ No

What is your experience with my type of cancer? _____
_____

Are you involved in any research?   ❏ Yes   ❏ No

What is your interpretation of my pathology report? _____
_____

What treatments do you recommend and why? *(Fill in the Treatment Options Worksheet on page 99.)*
_____

How many times have you performed this surgery? _____

What are the success rates with this surgery? _____
_____

What are the chances of removing all the cancer? _____
_____

Will there be scars or disfigurements?   ❏ Yes   ❏ No

What complications are associated with surgery? _____
_____

Will I require drain bulbs?   ❏ Yes   ❏ No   *(If yes, please see pages 102 & 103)*

How will I care for my surgical site? _____
_____

What should I know about pain management? _____
_____

What is the length of the operation & hospital stay? _____

What is the recuperation time? _____

Will I need any additional tests? _____
_____

Questions for the Surgeon

What will my follow-up care be like? _____

_____

What kind of node biopsy will you perform? _____

_____

What is my prognosis? _____

_____

Do you recommend genetic testing for me? _____ ❑ Yes ❑ No

Are you involved in any clinical trials or research projects? _____ ❑ Yes ❑ No

Am I a good candidate for participating in a trial? _____ ❑ Yes ❑ No
(If Yes, see Clinical Trial Questions on page 68).

Who else do you recommend I contact and why? _____

Where do you recommend I be treated and why? _____

How soon do I have to make a decision? _____

May I speak with other patients of yours? _____ ❑ Yes ❑ No

Will my insurance cover the costs? _____ ❑ Yes ❑ No

If not, are there financial assistance programs to help cover the costs? ❑ Yes ❑ No

Where can I get more information? _____

_____

What is the best way to communicate with you? _____

_____

Additional questions/comments: _____

_____

_____

_____

_____

Surgical Treatment Options

List the advantages and disadvantages of each option you are a candidate for.

Opinion given by: _____

Option: _____

Treatment length: _____ Odds of Cure: _____

Risks:_____

_____

_____

_____

Side effects: _____

_____

_____

_____

_____

Other factors: _____

_____

_____

_____

Option: _____

Treatment length: _____ Odds of Cure: _____

Risks:_____

_____

_____

_____

Side effects: _____

_____

_____

_____

Other factors: _____

_____

_____

_____

Surgical Treatment Options

List the advantages and disadvantages of each option you are a candidate for.

Opinion given by: _____

Option: _____

Treatment length: _____ Odds of Cure: _____

Risks:_____
_____
_____
_____
_____

Side effects: _____
_____
_____
_____
_____
_____

Other factors: _____
_____
_____
_____
_____

Option: _____

Treatment length: _____ Odds of Cure: _____

Risks:_____
_____
_____
_____
_____

Side effects: _____
_____
_____
_____
_____

Other factors: _____
_____
_____
_____

Pre-Operative Questions

What tests will I need before surgery?

❑ Pre-Admission Physical

❑ Chest X-ray

❑ Lab Work

❑ Other _____

Does my insurance provider cover everything? ❑ Yes ❑ No

If not, what is my responsibility? _____

Can I make special payment arrangements? ❑ Yes ❑ No

If yes, please explain: _____

_____

Do I need medication the night before? ❑ Yes ❑ No

If yes, please explain: _____

Where should I go on the day of surgery? _____

Should I take my regular medication on this day? ❑ Yes ❑ No

What should I wear? _____

When should I stop eating? _____

What should I bring? _____

What should I leave at home? _____

Where should my companion be during my surgery? _____

How will you contact them? _____

Can I have visitors? ❑ Yes ❑ No

Additional questions/comments: _____

_____

_____

Diagnosis: Breast Cancer 101

Drain Bulb Questions

How do I take care of my drains? _____

_____

Do I need someone to help me?   ❑ Yes   ❑ No

Will they hurt?   ❑ Yes   ❑ No

How do I measure the fluid? _____

_____

How do I clean them? _____

_____

What if they leak? _____

_____

What if they get clogged? _____

_____

How are they removed? _____

_____

What do I wear? _____

When can I shower or take a bath? _____

When can I wear a bra again? _____

_____

What are my restrictions? _____

_____

Can I move my arms? _____

Should I exercise?   ❑ Yes   ❑ No   If so, what kind? _____

_____

What should I report immediately? _____

_____

Additional questions/comments: _____

_____

_____

Drain Bulb Care

Measure and record the amount of fluid in each drain, and observe any changes in the fluid. Keeping accurate records will help your surgeon determine when to remove your bulbs.

Date	Time	Drain 1 Fluid Amount	Drain 2 Fluid Amount	Total Fluid Amount	Comments

Side Effects

Fill in the appropriate contact information for your treatment team and record any side effects you may be experiencing.

S: Surgery   **C:** Chemotherapy   **RS:** Reconstructive Surgery   **H:** Hormonal   **R:** Radiation
B: Biological   **M:** Medications   **CT:** Complementary therapy   **N:** Nutrition   **E:** Exercise

Contact	Name	Phone	Email
Surgeon			
Plastic Surgeon			
Radiologist			
Medical Oncologist			
Nurse Navigator			

Category	Side Effect/ Action Taken	Comments	Date	Time

Side Effects

Fill in the appropriate contact information for your treatment team and record any side effects you may be experiencing.

S: Surgery   **C:** Chemotherapy   **RS:** Reconstructive Surgery   **H:** Hormonal   **R:** Radiation

B: Biological   **M:** Medications   **CT:** Complementary therapy   **N:** Nutrition   **E:** Exercise

Contact	Name	Phone	Email
Surgeon			
Plastic Surgeon			
Radiologist			
Medical Oncologist			
Nurse Navigator			

Category	Side Effect/Action Taken	Comments	Date	Time

Surgery Follow-Up Questions

How do you feel the surgery went? _____

Were you able to remove all of the cancer?   ❑ Yes   ❑ No

   If not, what cancer remains? _____

_____

Were there any complications?   ❑ Yes   ❑ No

   If yes, please explain _____

_____

How long do I need to stay at the hospital? _____

What is my prognosis? _____

_____

How do I take care of the dressing on my incision? _____

_____

How much can I move my arm? _____

When can I shower? _____

_____

When do my stitches come out? _____

_____

How do I take care of my drains? (See Drain Bulb Questions on page 102) _____

_____

What symptoms should I call you about? _____

Do I need any prescriptions filled?   ❑ Yes   ❑ No

   If yes, what _____

_____

When should I see you again? _____

Who should I see next and when? _____

_____

Additional questions/comments: _____

_____

A woman is like a tea bag—you can't tell how strong she is until you put her in hot water.

- Eleanor Roosevelt

chapter
7

Post-Mastectomy Options

Exploring Your Options

Restoring your body image after a mastectomy can play a huge role in your emotional and physical recovery. The *Questions for the Plastic Surgeon* on page 114 and the *Post-Mastectomy Options Worksheet* on page 116 will help you navigate your options.

After a mastectomy you have three options: you can do nothing further, you can wear breast prostheses, or you can have breast reconstruction surgery. Many factors will go into your decision. Take your time and reflect on your emotions. Below are some questions to consider:

- How important are my breasts to me?

- How important are my breasts to my self-image and sexuality?

- Could I accept losing my breast(s)?

- Would I resent losing my breast(s)?

- How do I feel about radiation therapy?

- Would I rather wear prostheses than undergo surgery?

Doing Nothing Further

You may simply have had enough. The thought of more surgeries just doesn't appeal to you. You're not alone; many people are content to go no further than a mastectomy. The good news is that studies have shown people who choose to do nothing further feel equally as good as those who choose to have reconstructive surgery.

Wearing a Prosthesis

Breast prostheses (aka falsies) are professionally made artificial forms made out of foam or silicone that are shaped like breasts and inserted inside your bra. They come in all colors, shapes, and sizes. There are a number of ways you can buy them, from specialty shops to online shopping.

Patients often receive temporary soft prostheses before they leave the hospital. When your incision has healed, your doctor will give you a prescription for a permanent prosthesis. Some insurance policies will cover either prostheses or reconstructive surgery (not both), so you will want to check with your insurance provider regarding your coverage.

Breast Reconstruction

Then again, you can just decide to start over and rebuild. This option involves some type of breast reconstruction surgery that uses either your own tissue (autologous) or artificial material (implants) to rebuild a natural-looking breast. Reconstructive surgery is available for almost any woman who chooses to have a mastectomy. If you are considering reconstructive surgery, let your breast surgeon know. The type of initial surgery to remove your tumor can impact your reconstructive choices. Together, you and your surgeon will determine which kind of surgery is best for you.

> When facing breast surgery and reconstruction, I found it extremely helpful to speak to women who had had the same procedures that I was deciding on. Women who have gone through that particular surgical experience can give you their thoughts on the recovery you will be facing as well as how they are feeling about their surgical decision years later. Some will even be willing to show you their new boobs.
>
> – Judy H.

Implants

Breast implants are a rubberlike silicone shell or sack that are filled with saline or silicone gel and designed to recreate your breast following a mastectomy. Both saline and silicone implants are FDA- (Federal Drug Administration) approved for breast reconstruction use. Different factors will determine the appropriate type of implant reconstruction for you. These include but are not limited to: prior surgery, radiation history, breast size, and reconstructive goals.

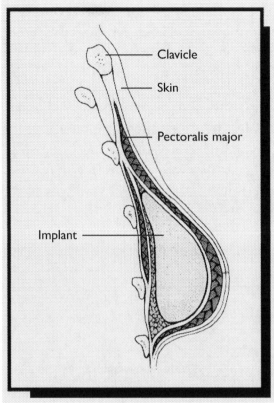

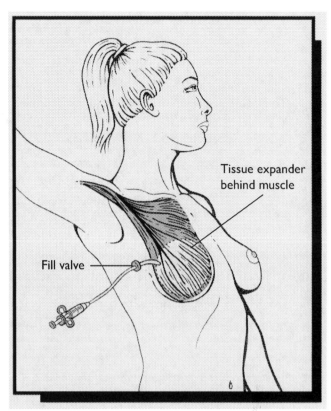

Figure 7.1   *Figure 7.2*

Breast implants are placed behind the chest (pectoralis) muscle in order to replace the tissue that has been removed. *(See Figure 7.1)* In most cases, the surgeon will create additional space behind the chest muscle in order to make room for your new breast implant. This can be achieved by placing a temporary adjustable implant, often referred to as a **tissue expander.**

Gradually, over several months, the tissue expander is injected with saline in order to stretch the skin. Once enough space has been created, the temporary implant is exchanged for a permanent one. Some people do not require the expansion process and are candidates for immediate placement of the permanent implant. However, most people will require a temporary expandable implant for one reason or another. *(See Figure 7.2)*

Autologous Reconstruction

In autologous (or flap) reconstruction, a new breast is shaped from tissue that is taken from other areas of the body such as the abdomen, back, buttocks, or thigh. Types of flap procedures to choose from are:

- **Pedicle flap** surgery involves removing muscle, skin, and fat from your donor site (the abdomen or back) while leaving the blood vessels attached during the transfer to the breast area. The tissue that was removed is transferred underneath your skin through a "tunnel" to your breast area while retaining its original blood supply.

- **Free-flap** surgery involves removing muscle, skin and fat from your donor site and detaching the blood vessels. The removed tissue is placed directly into an opening in the breast area, where the surgeon carefully reattaches the cut blood vessels to the new blood vessels under the armpit or in the chest wall.

- **Perforator flap** surgery involves removing only skin, fat, and smaller blood vessels (perforators) from the donor site, leaving the underlying muscle intact. The donor tissue is transferred to the breast area and reattached using microsurgery. Although this type of surgery takes longer than free-flap, the minimal impact on the donor site muscle function significantly reduces post-operative pain and length of hospital stay.

Abdominal Tissue Reconstruction Procedures

The most common donor site for breast reconstruction is the abdominal region. Three types of surgery are performed using tissue from the abdomen:

- **TRAM (Transverse Rectus Abdominus Myocutaneous flap):** This is the most common autologous flap used and works well for those women with additional abdominal fat. The surgeon takes the skin, fat, and transverse rectus abdominus myocutaneous muscle from the lower abdomen, along with its own blood supply (pedicle flap), and tunnels in underneath your upper abdomen to the chest area, where a new breast is formed. *(See Figure 7.3)*

- **DIEP (Deep Inferior Epigastric Perforator flap):** This procedure uses only abdominal skin and fat without the muscle and the deep inferior epigastric artery and vein and its perforators.

- **SIEA (Superficial Inferior Epigastric Artery flap):** This procedure uses abdominal skin, fat, and the superficial inferior epigastric artery and vein and its perforators. This perforator flap is disconnected from its original blood supply and is reconnected to the blood supply in the chest.

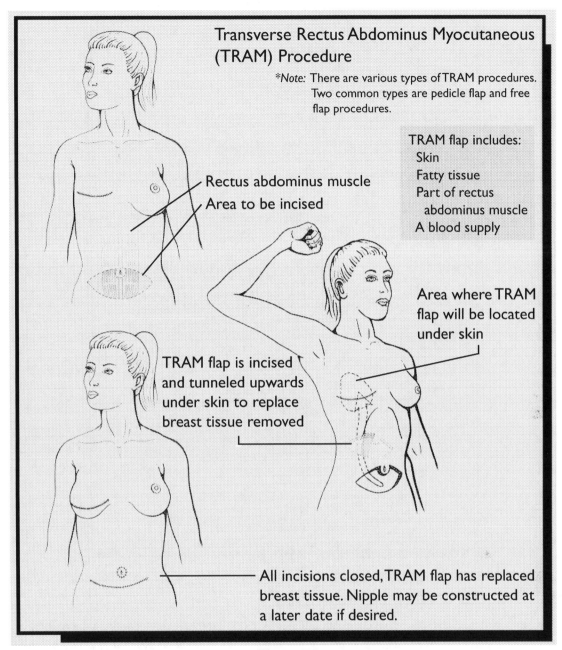

Transverse Rectus Abdominus Myocutaneous (TRAM) Procedure

Note: There are various types of TRAM procedures. Two common types are pedicle flap and free flap procedures.

TRAM flap includes:
Skin
Fatty tissue
Part of rectus abdominus muscle
A blood supply

Rectus abdominus muscle
Area to be incised

Area where TRAM flap will be located under skin

TRAM flap is incised and tunneled upwards under skin to replace breast tissue removed

All incisions closed, TRAM flap has replaced breast tissue. Nipple may be constructed at a later date if desired.

Figure 7.3

Back Tissue Reconstruction Procedures

Two procedures for breast reconstruction using tissue from the back are:

- **LD (Latissimus Dorsi muscle flap):** This type of surgery gets its name from the back muscle, the latissimus dorsi, which is removed along with skin, fat, and original blood supply (pedicle flap) from the back and used to create a new breast. Since the latissimus dorsi muscle in not large enough to build an entire breast for most women, an implant is commonly placed beneath it. (*See Figure 7.4*)

- **TAP (Thoracodorsal Artery Perforator flap):** This type of perforator flap surgery does not use the latissimus dorsi muscle but uses the skin and fat around this muscle to reconstruct the breast.

111

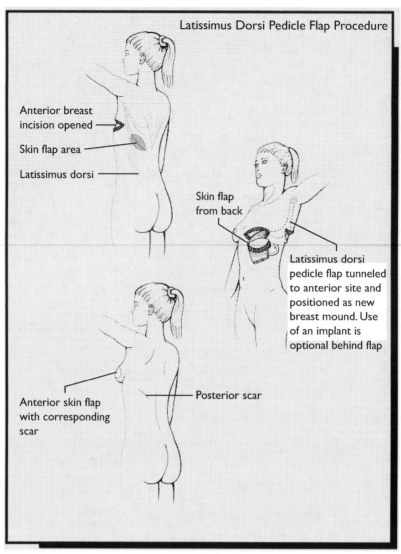

Latissimus Dorsi Pedicle Flap Procedure

Anterior breast
incision opened

Skin flap area

Latissimus dorsi

Skin flap
from back

Latissimus dorsi
pedicle flap tunneled
to anterior site and
positioned as new
breast mound. Use
of an implant is
optional behind flap

Anterior skin flap
with corresponding
scar

Posterior scar

Figure 7.4

Buttock Tissue Reconstruction Procedures

Two reconstruction techniques using tissue from the buttocks are perforator flap procedures. They use either the upper (superior) or lower (inferior) buttock skin and fat. **Both of these flaps are perforator flaps that require the use of microsurgery.** These are often abbreviated as SGAP (Superior Gluteal Artery Perforator flap) and IGAP (Inferior Gluteal Artery Perforator flap). (See *Figure 7.5*)

Nipple and Areola Reconstruction

If your nipple was removed, you have the option of having a nipple and areola recreated once you have healed from surgery. Your surgeon can construct a new nipple using existing skin and fat on the breast itself, using tissue from another area (such as the inner thigh), or using an artificial implant. The tissue is then molded into the shape of a nipple and attached to the breast mound. The areola (the colored area of tissue where the nipple sits) can be reconstructed by tattooing the area using a dye that matches the color of your other areola. Not all women have their nipples and areolas reconstructed. This is up to you.

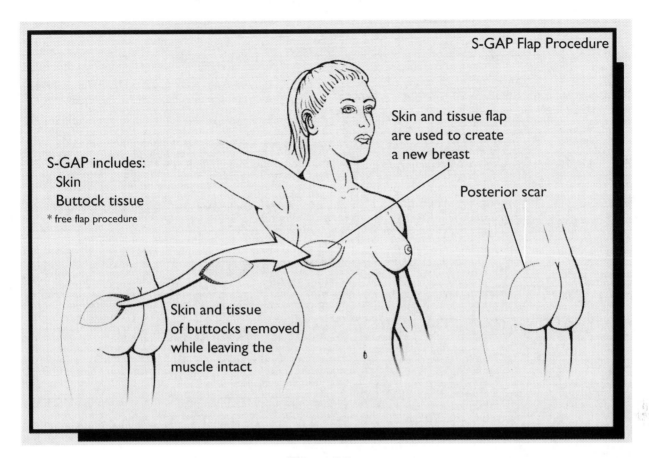

S-GAP Flap Procedure

Skin and tissue flap are used to create a new breast

Posterior scar

S-GAP includes:
Skin
Buttock tissue
* free flap procedure

Skin and tissue of buttocks removed while leaving the muscle intact

Figure 7.5

Choosing Your Reconstructive Surgeon

Before scheduling any consultation, call ahead and ask which treatments and procedures the doctor offers. Make sure you find a plastic surgeon that provides a full range of reconstruction options. If your choices are limited, move on to your next referral. You shouldn't be steered toward one surgical option simply because a doctor does not perform others.

Potential Side Effects and Follow-Up Care

After any major surgery, it takes time to adjust and get back to "your usual self." You may want to have someone with you at follow-up appointments with your surgeon. You most likely will not feel up to asking questions. Use the *Reconstruction Follow-Up Questions* on page 118 to keep track of what you need to do. Remember to ask which side effects you should report immediately and whom you should call. Use the *Side Effects Worksheet* on page 104 to record any reactions and ask for a copy of your surgery information to record on the *Treatment Summary Worksheet* on page 177.

Questions for the Plastic Surgeon

Are you board certified? ❑ Yes ❑ No

What is your experience with my type of cancer? _____

_____

Am I a good candidate for reconstructive surgery? ❑ Yes ❑ No

What types of surgery do you recommend for me and why? *(Fill in Post-Mastectomy Options Worksheet on page 116)* _____

_____

_____

Do you suggest implants or the use of my own body tissue? _____

_____

What kind of implants do you recommend and why? _____

_____

How many times have you performed each type of surgery? _____

When is the best time for me to have reconstruction? _____ ❑ Now ❑ Later

Why: _____

What if I need radiation therapy? _____

_____

What is the chance of infection and/or rejection with an implant device? _____

_____

Will you reconstruct my nipple and areola? ❑ Yes ❑ No

What kind of feeling will I have in my reconstructed breast? _____

_____

Will my breast be hard or soft when touched? _____

How does this surgery affect my odds of recurrence? _____

How many surgeries will I need? _____

Questions for the Plastic Surgeon

How many surgeries require hospitalization? _____

What will I look like after surgery? _____

How will my new breast compare with my other breast? _____

Will anything need to be done to my other breast? _____

What is my expected recovery time? _____

Will surgery limit my activities? _____

What if I am unhappy with the results? _____

May I see pictures of other patients who have had the same surgery? _____

_____

May I speak with other patients of yours?   ❏ Yes   ❏ No

What will my follow-up care be? _____

Will I need at-home care?   ❏ Yes   ❏ No

What is the best way to communicate with you? _____

How soon do I have to make a decision? _____

If I don't choose surgery what prostheses are available? _____

Will my insurance cover the costs? _____

If not, are there financial assistance programs to help cover the costs?   ❏ Yes   ❏ No

Where can I get more information? _____

What is the best way to communicate with you? _____

Additional questions/comments: _____

_____

_____

_____

_____

Post-Mastectomy Options

List the advantages and disadvantages of each option you are a candidate for.

Opinion given by: _____

Option: _____

Treatment length: _____ Odds of Cure: _____

Risks:_____
_____
_____
_____

Side effects: _____
_____
_____
_____
_____

Other factors: _____
_____
_____
_____

Option: _____

Treatment length: _____ Odds of Cure: _____

Risks:_____
_____
_____
_____

Side effects: _____
_____
_____
_____

Other factors: _____
_____
_____
_____

Post-Mastectomy Options

List the advantages and disadvantages of each option you are a candidate for.

Opinion given by: _____

Option: _____

Treatment length: _____ Odds of Cure: _____

Risks:_____

_____

_____

_____

Side effects: _____

_____

_____

_____

_____

Other factors: _____

_____

_____

_____

Option: _____

Treatment length: _____ Odds of Cure: _____

Risks:_____

_____

_____

_____

Side effects: _____

_____

_____

_____

_____

Other factors: _____

_____

_____

_____

Reconstruction Follow-Up Questions

How do you feel the surgery went? _____

Were you able to remove all of the cancer? ❑ Yes ❑ No

    If not, what cancer remains?_____

Were there any complications? ❑ Yes ❑ No

    If yes, please explain _____

_____

How long do I need to stay at the hospital? _____

What is my prognosis? _____

_____

How do I take care of the dressing on my incision? _____

_____

How much can I move my arm? _____

When can I shower? _____

_____

When do my stitches come out? _____

_____

How do I take care of my drains? (See *Drain Bulb Questions* on page 102)_____

_____

What symptoms should I call you about? _____

Do I need any prescriptions filled? ❑ Yes ❑ No

    If yes, what_____

_____

When should I see you again? _____

Who should I see next and when? _____

_____

Additional questions/comments: _____

_____

_____

*The best way out is
always through.*

- Robert Frost

chapter 8

Radiation Strategies

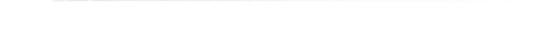

Exploring Your Options

Surgery alone may not be enough to effectively treat your cancer. It depends on what type of cancer you have and what other treatments you are exploring. If it turns out that radiation therapy is in your best interest, the *Questions for the Radiation Oncologist* on page 124 and the *Radiation Options Worksheet* on page 126 can help you in your decision-making process.

Standard operating procedure for a broken bone or even a cavity is an x-ray. Some forms of **radiation therapy,** also known as **radiotherapy,** use the same high-energy radiation from x-rays, only stronger, while other types may use gamma rays, neutrons, or protons to kill cancer cells and shrink tumors. Radiation therapy can either directly damage cancer cells' DNA (the molecules within the cell that carry genetic information) or create charged particles within the cancer cells; this in turn destroys their ability to reproduce. When the damaged cells die, they are eliminated naturally by the body.

Radiation therapy given during surgery is called **intraoperative radiation therapy (IORT).** IORT is currently being explored to deliver a single high dose of intraoperative radiation therapy immediately following lumpectomy with promising results in recent studies. IORT is sometimes used when external-beam radiation is not an option due to the location of the tumor.

Radiation Therapy and Implants

If you already have breast implants, you may face cosmetic issues. Radiation can increase fibrosis or scarring around the implant and can alter its shape and size. Additional surgery might be needed to correct the look of the breast.

If you are considering implants after a mastectomy you will want to discuss the risks with your radiation oncologist and reconstructive surgeon. The skin after radiation can be stiffer and thinner, making implants a less desirable choice. Sometimes, following a mastectomy, reconstructive surgeons place a temporary skin expander that remains in place during the radiation treatments. The permanent implant is then placed following completion of radiation therapy.

Types of Radiation Treatments

Radiation delivered by a machine outside the body is called **external-beam radiation therapy.** Radiation delivered by radioactive material placed in the body near cancer cells is called **internal radiation** or **brachytherapy**, and may also be referred to as partial breast radiation. Another form of treatment known as **systemic radiation therapy** uses a radioactive substance that is administered by pill or injection and travels in the blood to tissues throughout the body.

External Radiation

External-beam therapy is often delivered by a machine called a **linear accelerator.** (*See Figure 8.1*) This machine uses targeted high-energy x-rays (photons) to kill any remaining cancer cells and stop them from spreading. The radiation is delivered through highly precise beams aimed at the tumor and an area of tissue surrounding it.

In the case of breast cancer, radiation is either directed to the whole breast or partial breast, encompassing the surgical site. It is given in tangents, or angles, so that it travels through the breast and out into the air, limiting the exposure to surrounding organs like the heart and lungs. The radiation is the same as that used in x-rays, only stronger. The procedure is painless, but often is accompanied by side effects.

I learned a few tricks along the way during my radiation treatments. If you wear a wig, wear a button-up shirt to treatments. It makes it much easier to keep your hair on.

Ditch wearing your bra as soon as you get home from work to keep it from rubbing against you. Last but not least, Vitamin E capsules work great to soothe skin irritation.

–Cara N.

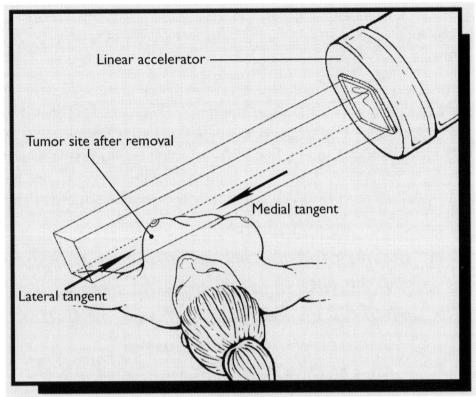

Linear accelerator

Tumor site after removal

Medial tangent

Lateral tangent

Figure 8.1

Internal Radiation

Another form of therapy is **internal radiation** or **brachytherapy,** which can be delivered by **interstitial** or **intracavitary** techniques. This method temporarily implants a source of radiation directly into the tumor or surgical site in order to wipe out any remaining cancer cells. The radiation implant could be seeds, catheters, or a small soft balloon that delivers radiation by a computer-controlled machine. Treatment duration varies based on the method of delivery.

Areas Treated

Radiation may be given as whole breast irradiation (WBI), accelerated hypofractionated radiation radiotherapy (AHF-RT) or as accelerated partial breast irradiation (APBI).

- **WBI** is given to your entire breast, and is generally expanded to cover your chest wall and a majority of the underarm (axillary) area. It usually requires twenty-five treatments, given daily Monday through Friday for five to six weeks. Each treatment delivers a low dose of radiation that kills cancer cells and affects healthy cells as well. At the end of the therapy, you may be given more radiation, called a boost, to the part of the breast that had the tumor to help get rid of any cancer left in the area. Your boost radiation session may be similar to a regular external radiation session or you may be given some form of internal radiation. If you have multiple positive lymph nodes, radiation may also be delivered to regional lymph node areas such as the lower neck above the clavicle bone.

- **AHF-RT** delivers higher doses of external radiation to the whole breast in fewer treatments than traditional radiation therapy. Treatments may be given over the course of three weeks.

- **APBI** delivers a highly effective dose of radiation to the partial breast surgical site while greatly reducing treatment time. It may be administered by external beam radiation or internally via brachytherapy, using a specialized catheter (flexible tube) that is inserted into the cavity left behind after removal of the tumor. A radioactive iridium seed is placed within the device under computer control to kill breast cancer cells that may remain after surgery.

The timing of radiation therapy is important, especially if you are considering reconstructive breast surgery. Be sure to discuss this with both your radiation oncologist and your surgeon.

Beginning Radiation Treatment

The Planning Session

Since radiation can cause damage to normal tissue, it must be carefully planned and precisely administered in the correct location. If you have decided to have external-beam therapy, you will need to schedule a planning session in which your treatments are "simulated" in order to create an accurate map of how and where the radiation will be delivered.

During the simulation you will be working with the radiation oncologist and technicians, who will give you small marks on your skin. These marks, about the size of a freckle, are used to make sure you are correctly positioned for each treatment. The marks might be ink spots or permanent tattoos. If they are ink spots, it is important not to wash them off until after you finish your radiation therapy. The simulation will last about an hour and is generally done with the aid of a CT scanner. You will lie on the table with your arms above your head while the oncologist calculates the proper dose of radiation and the best areas to receive it.

I was fortunate enough to find a caring professional who went to great pains to see that I was comfortable and never in any danger of radiation burns.

It should be stressed to people that there sometimes is a great tiredness and lethargy that comes with radiation, and they should allow for this to last for at least three to four months.

—Bette H.

Treatment Days

Don't worry if you are claustrophobic. There is plenty of open space between you and the machine. For treatment you will undress from the waist up and change into a gown. You will lie on a table with the linear accelerator machine above it. Each session lasts around ten to twenty minutes. Most of this time is spent positioning your body with a head and armrest. Sometimes positioning your arm after you have had surgery can be a little uncomfortable, but for the most part, treatments are painless.

Treatment Tips

The following tips can help you through your radiation treatments. Ask your doctor for further recommendations.

- Wear clothing that is easy to take off.

- Avoid extremes of hot or cold on your skin.

- Do not use deodorants or deodorant soaps.

- Wear loose-fitting, soft cotton clothing and bras.

- Ask your doctor or technician what lotions you may use.

- Keep the treated area out of the sun.

- Do not shave under your arms with a razor blade.

- Use reliable birth control, since radiation can harm a fetus.

> **The colder the x-ray table, the more of your body is required to be on it.**
>
> —*Steven Wright*

Potential Side Effects

Radiation therapy does not kill cancer cells immediately. This is why treatment often takes days or weeks to complete. Side effects usually start to appear two to three weeks after starting treatments. Be sure to ask your technician or doctor what side effects to expect and what you should report immediately. The *Side Effects Worksheet* on page 104 will help you keep track of any reactions.

Ending Treatments

Remember to talk with your radiation oncologist about your follow-up care (using the *Radiation Follow-Up Questions* on page 128) and to get a copy of your treatment summary report to record on the *Treatment Summary Worksheet* on page 177.

Questions for the Radiation Oncologist

Why are you recommending radiation therapy for me? _____
_____

How does this treatment improve my prognosis and chance of recurrence? _____
_____

What are the advantages and disadvantages? *(See page 126)* _____
_____

How does radiation therapy affect other treatment options? _____
_____

What are the short-term side effects? _____
_____

How long might they last? _____

What are the long-term side effects/risks? _____
_____

How can I prevent or treat these side effects? _____
_____

Which side effects should I report to you immediately? _____
_____

How soon should radiation therapy be started? _____

In what form and how often will I get the treatment? _____
_____

Will the whole breast or partial breast be treated? _____

How long will each treatment take and how many treatments will I have? _____
_____

What clothes should I wear to the therapy sessions? _____
_____

Will I need someone to go with me?　❑ Yes　❑ No

Questions for the Radiation Oncologist

How will you evaluate the effectiveness of my treatment? _____
_____

How will treatments affect my daily life? _____
_____

Can I exercise during treatment? _____

Are there special precautions I should take while having radiation therapy, or afterwards?
_____
_____

Will treatments affect my sex life? _____

What lotion, soaps, or other skincare products should I use or avoid? _____
_____

What do I need to consider if I would like to have a child after breast cancer treatment?
_____
_____
_____

May I speak with other patients of yours?   ❑ Yes   ❑ No

Will the cost of the treatment be covered by my health insurance?   ❑ Yes   ❑ No

If not, are there financial assistance programs to help cover the costs?   ❑ Yes   ❑ No

Where can I get more information? _____

What is the best way to communicate with you? _____

Additional questions/comments: _____
_____
_____

Radiation Options

List the advantages and disadvantages of each option you are a candidate for.

Opinion given by: _____

Option: _____

Treatment length: _____ Odds of Cure: _____

Risks:_____
_____
_____
_____

Side effects: _____
_____
_____
_____
_____

Other factors: _____
_____
_____
_____

Option: _____

Treatment length: _____ Odds of Cure: _____

Risks:_____
_____
_____
_____

Side effects: _____
_____
_____
_____

Other factors: _____
_____
_____
_____

workingoutcancer.com

Radiation Options

List the advantages and disadvantages of each option you are a candidate for.

Opinion given by: _____

Option: _____

Treatment length: _____ Odds of Cure: _____

Risks: _____

_____

_____

_____

Side effects: _____

_____

_____

_____

_____

Other factors: _____

_____

_____

_____

Option: _____

Treatment length: _____ Odds of Cure: _____

Risks: _____

_____

_____

_____

Side effects: _____

_____

_____

_____

Other factors: _____

_____

_____

_____

Radiation Follow-Up Questions

How am I doing? _____
_____
_____

Am I responding to the treatments as you had hoped? _____
_____
_____

What should I look out for? _____
_____
_____

What are my next steps? _____
_____
_____

What should I report to you? _____
_____
_____

When do I see you again? _____
_____

Who do I see next? _____
_____

Additional questions/comments: _____
_____
_____
_____
_____
_____
_____
_____
_____
_____
_____

> *Learn from yesterday,*
> *live for today,*
> *hope for tomorrow.*
>
> *- Albert Einstein*

chapter 9

Hormone and Targeted Therapies

Exploring Your Options

When you were first diagnosed, your cells were checked for certain hormone receptors and HER-2/neu. Depending on the results of those tests, you may be a candidate for hormonal and/or targeted therapy. The *Questions for the Medical Oncologist* on page 131 and the *Hormone and Targeted Therapy Options Worksheet* on page 133 will help you in making your treatment decisions.

What Is Hormone Therapy?

At some point or another, everyone seems to blame their mood swings on their **hormones,** the substances that aid in regulating your body functions. The two hormones that are involved in breast cancer are **estrogen** and **progesterone.** Estrogen (ER) is produced primarily by the ovaries and aids in developing female sex organs as well as regulating monthly menstrual cycles. Progesterone (PR) is released by the ovaries during each menstrual cycle to help prepare a woman's body for pregnancy and breastfeeding.

Receptors are the molecules on the surface of cells that recognize hormones circulating in the blood stream. In certain breast cancers, hormones can attach to the cancer cell receptors and increase their ability to multiply. In these situations, **hormone therapy** is a treatment given to block the body's naturally occurring estrogen and prevent the cancer from growing.

Do not confuse the terms "hormone therapy" and "hormone replacement therapy." Hormone therapy for cancer treatment stops hormones from getting to breast cancer cells. Hormone replacement therapy, sometimes used for post-menopausal women, adds more hormones to the body to counter the effects of menopause.

Types of Hormone Therapy

Hormone therapy for breast cancer may be achieved by drugs or surgery. Your medical oncologist can prescribe drugs that either block estrogen and/or progesterone from promoting breast cancer cell growth, or that prevent your body from making estrogen.

- **Tamoxifen** is a drug that stops estrogen from binding to its receptor and is given to pre-menopausal or post-menopausal women.

- **Aromatase inhibitors** are drugs that prevent fat, muscle cells, and the adrenal glands from producing estrogen in post-menopausal women. They stop an enzyme called aromatase from turning other hormones into estrogen.

- **Pituitary down-regulators** are drugs that reduce the production of estrogen-stimulating hormones by the brain and are given to pre-menopausal women.

Depending on the type of cancer, some women who have not gone through menopause will require an ovarian ablation. This is a type of surgery to remove the ovaries, which are the body's main source of estrogen. This can also be achieved through radiation.

What Is Targeted Therapy?

When you aim at a target you want to hit the bull's eye. That's exactly what **targeted therapy** does. Targeted therapies are drugs that are aimed directly at the gene changes in cells that cause cancer. Cancers that test positive for HER-2/neu, a gene that is responsible for making HER-2 proteins and tend to be more aggressive and grow faster, can respond to targeted therapy. The therapy works by taking advantage of your body's own immune system—which defends the body against infections and other disease—to act on cancer cells with little harm to your healthy cells.

Potential Side Effects and Follow-Up

These therapies often involve side effects. Ask your doctor what side effects to expect and which ones you should report immediately. Use the *Side Effect Worksheet* on page 104 to help keep track of any reactions. Discuss the length of your treatments and the appropriate follow-up care with your medical oncologist using the *Hormone/Targeted Therapy Follow-Up Questions* on page 135.

Questions for the Medical Oncologist

What is your experience with my type of cancer? _____

_____

Which therapies do you recommend for me and why? _____

_____

How does this treatment affect my prognosis and chances of recurrence? _____

_____

What are the short-term side effects? How long might they last? _____

_____

What are the long-term side effects/risks? _____

_____

How can I prevent or treat these side effects? _____

_____

Which side effects should I report to you immediately? _____

_____

How soon should this treatment be started? _____

_____

In what form and how often will I get treatments? _____

How long will I be on this therapy? _____

How will you evaluate the effectiveness of my therapy? _____

_____

How will treatments affect my daily life? _____

_____

Is there a generic form of this hormone/biological treatment? ☐ Yes ☐ No

Is it as effective as the name brand? ☐ Yes ☐ No

Will I take the hormone/biological therapy along with my other treatments? ☐ Yes ☐ No

Questions for the Medical Oncologist

What do I need to consider if I would like to have a child after treatment? _____

_____

Will the cost of the treatment be covered by my health insurance?   ❑ Yes ❑ No

If not, are there financial assistance programs that will help cover the costs?   ❑ Yes ❑ No

Will I need more tests or exams?   ❑ Yes ❑ No

If so, which tests and how often will they be needed?   _____

_____

What are the risks if I stop taking the therapy?   _____

_____

May I speak with other patients of yours?   ❑ Yes ❑ No

Where can I get more information?   _____

What is the best way to communicate with you?   _____

Additional questions/comments: _____

_____

_____

_____

_____

_____

_____

_____

_____

_____

_____

_____

workingoutcancer.com

Questions for the Medical Oncologist

Hormone and Targeted Therapy Options

List the advantages and disadvantages of each option you are a candidate for.

Opinion given by: _____

Option: _____

Treatment length: _____ Odds of Cure: _____

Risks:_____
_____
_____
_____

Side effects: _____
_____
_____
_____
_____

Other factors: _____
_____
_____
_____

Option: _____

Treatment length: _____ Odds of Cure: _____

Risks:_____
_____
_____
_____

Side effects: _____
_____
_____
_____

Other factors: _____
_____
_____
_____

Hormone and Targeted Therapy Options

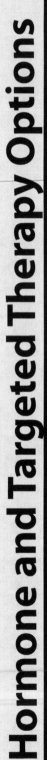
Hormone and Targeted Therapy Options

List the advantages and disadvantages of each option you are a candidate for.

Opinion given by: _____

Option: _____

Treatment length: _____ Odds of Cure: _____

Risks:_____
_____
_____
_____

Side effects: _____
_____
_____
_____
_____

Other factors: _____
_____
_____
_____

Option: _____

Treatment length: _____ Odds of Cure: _____

Risks:_____
_____
_____
_____

Side effects: _____
_____
_____
_____

Other factors: _____
_____
_____
_____

Hormone/Targeted Therapy Follow-Up Questions

How am I doing? _____
_____
_____

Am I responding to the treatments as you had hoped? _____
_____
_____

What should I look out for? _____
_____
_____

What are my next steps? _____
_____
_____

What should I report to you? _____
_____
_____

When do I see you again? _____
_____

Who do I see next? _____
_____

Additional questions/comments: _____
_____
_____
_____
_____
_____
_____
_____
_____
_____
_____

Notes

Diagnosis: Breast Cancer

> *Determination gives you the resolve to keep going in spite of the roadblocks that lay before you.*
>
> *- Denis Waitley*

chapter **10**

Chemotherapy

Exploring Your Options

Chemotherapy is a scary-sounding word, but it doesn't need to be. Chemotherapy drugs have come a long way and many side effects are completely manageable. Can it be intense? Yes. Are you going to lose your hair? Maybe. Your side effects will depend on the type of cancer you have and what chemotherapy you need. Use the *Chemotherapy Questions* on page 143 and the *Chemotherapy Options Worksheet* on page 145 when you meet with the medical oncologist to help you in the decision-making process.

What Is Chemotherapy?

Chemotherapy, often referred to as **chemo,** uses chemicals (drugs) to kill or disable cancer cells that are growing and dividing in your body. It's often used to prevent the cancer from spreading, slow its growth, relieve painful symptoms, and achieve long-term remission.

When chemotherapy is used to shrink the tumor before breast surgery it is referred to as neo-adjuvant chemotherapy. When it's given after breast surgery it is called adjuvant therapy. If you have metastatic cancer (cancer that has spread from the breast to other parts of the body), chemotherapy is used to disable cancer cells, reduce cancer-related symptoms, and prolong your survival.

Many different drugs are used in numerous combinations to treat breast cancer. Many factors will determine which chemotherapy drugs are best suited for treating your type of breast cancer. Together, you and your medical oncologist will discuss which drugs are appropriate for you.

How Is Chemotherapy Administered?

Chemotherapy drugs are most often injected into a vein by an IV (intravenous line). Sometimes a permanent IV device (called a port or port-a-cath) or a pump is used for the duration of your treatments. A port is a device that is surgically inserted under the skin, usually on the chest opposite the side of your surgery. Treatments usually are administered in a clinic, at a hospital, or at your doctor's office by a certified oncology nurse.

> **I was going to buy a book on hair loss, but the pages kept falling out.**
>
> —*Jay London*

Chemotherapy Scheduling

How long is all of this going to take? It depends on your type of cancer. Treatment plans deliver specific chemotherapy drugs at precise doses and intervals. These are called scheduled cycles. Cycling allows the cancer cells to be attacked at their most vulnerable times and gives your body a chance to recover between treatments.

- **Cycle duration:** Chemotherapy treatments use either a single drug or a combination of drugs. Treatments can last minutes, hours, or days, depending on the protocol.

- **Cycle frequency:** Chemotherapy may be administered weekly, biweekly, every three weeks, or monthly. For example, a day of chemotherapy followed by three weeks off is classified as one cycle.

- **Cycle quantity:** The chemotherapy "regimen" refers to the duration of the chemotherapy from start to finish.

- **Cycle dose:** Dose-dense chemotherapy gives the prescribed amount (dose) of chemotherapy in a shorter period of time, potentially resulting in a higher dose per session.

Potential Side Effects

Believe it or not, side effects are a good thing. They mean that the chemotherapy is doing its job. Since chemotherapy works by killing only dividing cells, most of your side effects will occur because of the treatment's effect on the healthy cells in your body that are also constantly dividing. The areas commonly affected are:

- Bone marrow, resulting in lowered white blood cells (which fight infection), red blood cells (which carry oxygen), and platelets (which stop bleeding)

- Gastrointestinal tract, resulting in stomach pain, constipation and/or diarrhea

- Mouth mucous membranes, resulting in mouth sores

- Vaginal mucous membranes, resulting in vaginal dryness

- Hair follicles, resulting in hair loss

Your side effects will vary depending on your health and on the dosages and types of drugs you are using. Common drug therapies and their side effects are listed in Table 10.1.

Table 10.1: Common Chemotherapy Drugs for Breast Cancer	
Alkylators: Interfere with the cell's DNA and inhibits cancer cell growth.	
Cytoxan® (cyclophosphamide)	Lowered blood counts Hair loss Nausea/vomiting Loss of appetite Loss of menstruation Darkening of skin
Anthracyclines: Change the structure of cellular DNA	
Adriamycin® (doxorubicin) Ellence® (epirubicin)	Lowered blood counts Hair loss Nausea/vomiting Sore mouth Loss of appetite Diarrhea Changes in heart rhythm Changes in nail beds Sun sensitivity Loss of menstruation Red urine
Doxil® (doxorubicin HCI liposome)	Lowered blood counts Sore mouth Flaking or peeling of the skin Rash Swelling/pain

Continued on Next Page

Table 10.1: Common Chemotherapy Drugs for Breast Cancer, *continued*	
Taxanes: Prevent cancer cells from dividing	
Taxol® (pacilitaxel)	Hair loss Low white blood counts Muscle/joint pain Tingling or burning in hands and/or feet
Taxotere® (docetaxel)	Hair loss Low white blood counts Low platelet counts Diarrhea Excessive tearing Nail bed tenderness/damage Loss of appetite Nausea/vomiting Numbness and tingling in hands and feet Rash
Antimetabolites: Interfere with cancer cell division needed to make new DNA	
5-FU® (5 fluorouracil)	Some hair loss Low white blood counts Sore mouth Nail changes Diarrhea Loss of appetite Nausea/vomiting Rash Dark veins at injection site
Methotrexate®	Dizziness/drowsiness Headache Swollen, tender gums Loss of appetite Red eyes Hair loss
Antimitotic: Prevents cancer cells from dividing	
Navelbine®	Diarrhea/constipation Hair loss Low white blood count Nausea/vomiting Weakness Pain after treatment

[National Institutes of Health]

Ask your doctor what side effects to expect and which ones you should report immediately. Use the *Side Effects Worksheet* on page 104 to keep track of any reactions.

Beginning Chemotherapy Treatment

See Your Dentist

The health of your teeth and gums can affect your treatments. Taking care of your dental health before starting chemotherapy can help you ward off serious complications such as infection, which could possibly force your oncologist to delay treatment. Make an appointment to talk with your dentist and explain your situation. Chances are he or she has met and treated other patients under similar circumstances and will be well-equipped to assist you.

Treatment Supplies

Although everyone responds differently to chemotherapy, you can anticipate several common reactions. You may have been told that you will lose your hair. Emotionally, this can be a tough side effect. If you are planning to wear a wig, look for one before you lose your hair. Not only will you be prepared, you will have a better chance of matching your current hair style and color. You can take this opportunity to change colors or styles if you like. Hey, why not?

Many things can change during chemotherapy, such as how your mouth feels, the way food tastes, and your bowel habits. It can help to have the following items readily available:

> I was not prepared for how hard it was psychologically to be bald (or how cold my head would be). Every time I put my wig on I felt like an imposter. I scoured the Internet looking for hats or wigs.
>
> God bless YouTube, for it was here I found a video of another patient who had filmed the weekly progression of her hair growing back. I don't know who she is but she kept me going. I am eternally grateful to her for paying it forward.
>
> —Cara N.

- Oral rinse
- Hypoallergenic lotion
- Prilosec (or other heartburn medication)
- Wigs, scarves, and hats
- Doctor-recommended items

- Toothpaste for sensitive teeth
- Hats for sleeping
- Hand sanitizer
- Thermometer

Organizing Your Medicines

Your medicine cabinet will soon start to look like a full-blown pharmacy. It helps to organize your medicines and instructions into an easy-to-follow schedule. Your treatment cycle will most likely be divided into a pre-treatment phase, a treatment phase, and a post-treatment phase. Try color-coding your medicines for easy reference and using the *Chemotherapy Calendar Worksheets* on page 147.

What to Expect at Each Visit

You're going to spend a lot of time at your doctor's office getting poked and prodded. The average breast cancer chemotherapy visit lasts from one to six hours, including time with your medical and nursing teams. At each visit your blood counts will be checked and you will be weighed. You may also get anti-nausea medicines and other treatments to make your chemotherapy easier to tolerate. Keep track of your treatment sessions using the *Chemotherapy Sessions Worksheet* on page 148.

Ending Treatment

When your treatments are over you can use the *Chemotherapy Follow-Up Questions* on page 150 to discuss your results with your medical oncologist. Remember to obtain your treatment summary report for your records and record it on the *Treatment Summary Worksheet* on page 177.

Chemotherapy Questions

What is your experience with my type of cancer? _____
_____

Why is chemotherapy recommended for me? _____
_____

How does this treatment improve my prognosis? _____
_____

What are the names of the drugs I will take and why have you chosen them for me?
_____
_____
_____
_____
_____

What are the short–term side effects of this type of chemotherapy? _____
_____
_____
_____

What are the long-term side effects? _____
_____
_____
_____

How can I prevent or treat these side effects? _____
_____

How will they impact my daily life? _____
_____

Which side effects should I report to you immediately? _____
_____

Chemotherapy Questions

How soon should chemotherapy be started? _____

In what form and how often will I get the treatment? _____
_____

How long will each treatment take and how many treatments will I have? _____
_____

How will you evaluate the effectiveness of my treatment? _____
_____

Will I need someone to go with me?   ❏ Yes   ❏ No

How will treatments affect my daily life? _____
_____

Can I exercise during treatments? _____

Are there special precautions I should take while on chemotherapy or afterwards?
_____
_____
_____

Will the cost of the treatment be covered by my health insurance?   ❏ Yes   ❏ No

If not, are there financial assistance programs to help cover the costs?   ❏ Yes   ❏ No

What is the best way to communicate with you? _____

Where can I get more information? _____

Additional questions/comments: _____
_____
_____
_____
_____
_____

Chemotherapy Options

List the advantages and disadvantages of each option you are a candidate for.

Opinion given by: _____

Option: _____

Treatment length: _____ Odds of Cure: _____

Risks:_____
_____
_____
_____

Side effects: _____
_____
_____
_____
_____

Other factors: _____
_____
_____
_____

Option: _____

Treatment length: _____ Odds of Cure: _____

Risks:_____
_____
_____
_____

Side effects: _____
_____
_____
_____

Other factors: _____
_____
_____
_____

Chemotherapy Options

List the advantages and disadvantages of each option you are a candidate for.

Opinion given by: _____

Option: _____

Treatment length: _____ Odds of Cure: _____

Risks:_____
_____
_____
_____

Side effects: _____
_____
_____
_____
_____

Other factors: _____
_____
_____
_____

Option: _____

Treatment length: _____ Odds of Cure: _____

Risks:_____
_____
_____
_____

Side effects: _____
_____
_____
_____

Other factors: _____
_____
_____
_____

Chemotherapy Options

Chemotherapy Calendar

You may find it helpful to color code your medications for easy reference. Fill in the days and time you will need to take your medications.

Medicines:

1. _____ 4. _____ 7. _____

2. _____ 5. _____ 8. _____

3. _____ 6. _____ 9. _____

Week

Time	Monday	Tuesday	Wednesday	Thursday	Friday	Saturday	Sunday

Week

Time	Monday	Tuesday	Wednesday	Thursday	Friday	Saturday	Sunday

Chemotherapy Calendar

Chemotherapy Sessions

Your nurse or doctor can assist you in recording your information for each chemotherapy treatment.

Session Number:

Medication Name	Dose	How it was Given	Allergic Reactions	Side Effects

Weight: **Hemoglobin:**   **White Blood Count:**   **Platelets:**   **Tumor Marker:**

Notes/Comments

Session Number:

Medication Name	Dose	How it was Given	Allergic Reactions	Side Effects

Weight: **Hemoglobin:**   **White Blood Count:**   **Platelets:**   **Tumor Marker:**

Notes/Comments

Chemotherapy Sessions

Your nurse or doctor can assist you in recording your information for each chemotherapy treatment.

Session Number:

Medication Name	Dose	How it was Given	Allergic Reactions	Side Effects

Weight: Hemoglobin: White Blood Count: Platelets: Tumor Marker:

Notes/Comments

Session Number:

Medication Name	Dose	How it was Given	Allergic Reactions	Side Effects

Weight: Hemoglobin: White Blood Count: Platelets: Tumor Marker:

Notes/Comments

Chemotherapy Follow-Up Questions

How am I doing? _____
_____
_____

Am I responding to the treatments as you had hoped? _____
_____
_____

What should I look out for? _____
_____
_____

What are my next steps? _____
_____
_____

What should I report to you? _____
_____
_____

When do I see you again? _____
_____

Who do I see next? _____
_____

Additional questions/comments: _____
_____
_____
_____
_____
_____
_____
_____
_____
_____
_____

Chemotherapy Follow-Up Questions

Our food should be our medicine and our medicine should be our food.

- Hippocrates

Nutrition Strategies

Exploring Your Options

Athletes eat certain meals before big games for a reason. They are preparing their bodies to be at their best. You can do the same. Nutritional therapy involves looking at what you eat and developing a dietary plan to help control your side effects, lower your risk of infections, enhance your recovery time, and boost your strength and energy.

Since your nutritional needs will vary throughout your treatment, the simplest way for you to prepare is to use the *Questions for the Registered Dietician* on page 154 when meeting with a registered dietician to help form your nutrition game plan.

Treatment Tips

Here are some tips from the National Cancer Institute at the National Institutes of Health to help manage treatment-related side effects.

Taste Changes

- Eat small meals and snacks several times a day, eating when hungry

- Eat citrus (unless you have mouth sores)

- Eat high-protein foods

- Rinse your mouth before eating

- Use plastic utensils

- Have others prepare meals

Dry Mouth

- Increase your fluid intake

- Chew gum or suck on hard sugar-free candy

- Eat moist foods with sauces or gravies

- Eat frozen ice desserts

- Use a straw for liquids

There came a point for me when nothing was appealing to eat. Everything tasted wrong and there were times when I couldn't stand the look or smell or certain foods.

Then there was a period when eating was no problem, so I did so with gusto. What I wish I had known then was that the extra weight I would soon gain due to treatment-induced menopause was going to be very hard to lose. Ask for help with your food options. It will really make a difference in how you feel.

—Cara N.

Mouth Sores

- Eat soft, easy-to-swallow foods

- Avoid citrus fruits and spicy, salty, and rough foods

- Eat cold foods

- Use a blender for vegetables

- Practice good oral hygiene

- Use a mouth rinse such as Biotene

Dehydration

- Drink 8 to 12 cups of liquid a day

- Avoid drinks with caffeine like coffee, tea, and sodas

- Use anti-nausea medicines

- Drink between meals

Diarrhea
- Increase your potassium
- Drink plenty of fluids
- Avoid greasy food, high-fiber foods, and milk products

Constipation
- Increase fluids
- Increase fiber intake
- Exercise regularly

Low Blood Counts and Infections
- Wash hands often and rinse foods well
- Do not thaw foods at room temperature (use the refrigerator)
- Cook all foods thoroughly
- Avoid leftovers
- Check foods' expiration dates

Nausea
- Eat before treatments
- Eat dry foods
- Sip fluids slowly
- Rinse your mouth before and after eating
- Eat in a comfortable place, away from odors

> **Vegetarian... that's an old Indian word meaning "lousy hunter."**
> —*Andy Rooney*

Potential Side Effects

Some herbs and supplements, such as black cohosh, can interfere with chemotherapy drugs, other treatment medications, or radiation therapy. That's why it is very important to talk with your team about what food and supplements you are taking or considering using. Keep track of any reactions on the *Side Effects Worksheet* on page 104 and be sure to ask your doctor about what you should report immediately. Check in often with your dietician throughout your treatments and beyond to manage your changing nutritional needs.

Questions for the Registered Dietician

What should I eat before and after surgery? _____
_____
_____

How will the different proposed treatments affect my nutrition? _____
_____
_____
_____
_____
_____
_____

What should I do if I don't feel like eating? _____
_____
_____
_____

What can I do for mouth sores? _____
_____

What can I do for a dry mouth? _____
_____

What can I do for diarrhea? _____
_____

What can I do for constipation? _____
_____

What can I do for nausea/vomiting? _____
_____

What can I eat to increase my energy? _____
_____

Questions for the Registered Dietician

What should I eat to help with low blood counts or infections? _____

_____

_____

What can I eat to alleviate menopausal symptoms? _____

_____

What can I eat to protect my bone health? _____

_____

What can I eat to help with insomnia? _____

_____

What supplements/vitamins do you recommend and why? _____

_____

_____

What should I specifically avoid eating during my treatments? _____

_____

_____

May I speak with other patients of yours?   ❑ Yes   ❑ No

Will the cost of the treatment be covered by my health insurance?   ❑ Yes   ❑ No

If not, are there financial assistance programs to help cover the costs?   ❑ Yes   ❑ No

Additional questions/comments: _____

_____

_____

_____

_____

_____

_____

Notes

> *Those who think they have
> not time for bodily exercise
> will sooner or later have to
> find time for illness.*
>
> *- Edward Stanley*

chapter

12

Exercise Strategies

Exploring Your Options

Shouldn't you be allowed to take a break from exercise during treatments? Well, yes and no. Exercise plays a vital role in a successful treatment plan. There will be some days when it's okay to exercise, other days you may not be well enough. In fact, in 2010 the American College of Sports Medicine Round Table concluded that "exercise training is safe during and after cancer treatments and results in improvements in physical functioning, quality of life, and cancer-related fatigue in several cancer survivor groups."

Exercise can help relieve your treatment symptoms, shorten recovery times, boost your immune system and improve your mental attitude. Your exercise goals may be very similar to goals you had before your cancer diagnosis. However, this is not the time to train for a marathon or climb Mount Kilimanjaro.

It's also not the time to be a couch potato. You do need to move. Discuss with your treatment team when and how much you should exercise. One of your best resources will be a certified cancer exercise specialist. If you can't find one in your area refer to the Additional Resources in Section III. Use the *Questions for the Exercise Specialist* on page 160 to help develop your exercise plan.

Types of Exercise

The main types of exercise are:

- **Aerobic fitness:** This type of therapy focuses on physical activities that provide increased oxygen to the body, strengthening the heart and lungs. Walking is the most-often recommended aerobic exercise during treatment.

- **Flexibility:** This type of therapy focuses on the ability to move your joints through their full range of motion. It is especially important to regain flexibility after surgery.

- **Muscular endurance:** This type of therapy focuses on your muscles' ability to work continuously over a long period of time. Do not start any resistance training program until you have regained your full range of motion.

Whether you are new to exercise or have been doing it for years, check in with your treatment team to get medical clearance before you begin. Keep track of your exercise using the *Exercise Log Worksheet* on page 161

Exercise Tips:

- Start out slowly and gradually increase the amount of time you exercise.

- Pay close attention to how you feel.

- Gradually increase your exercising heart rate.

- Make sure you stay well-hydrated by drinking plenty of water.

- Try to build up to walking for 20 to 45 minutes four or five days each week.

- Work on the range of motion in your arms daily.

> **Whenever I feel the urge to exercise I lie down until it passes.**
>
> —*Mark Twain*

Potential Side Effects

Although there are specific risks associated with cancer treatments to consider when you exercise, consistent evidence shows that exercise is safe during and after cancer treatment and can potentially reduce the risk of (or delay) a recurrence.

There are certain times when exercise is not recommended. Do not exercise if you are experiencing:

- Low blood counts

- Fever

- Nausea or vomiting

- Muscle or joint pain or swelling

- Bleeding

- Dizziness

Ask your treatment team what you should be on the lookout for. If you experience any negative reactions be sure to record them on the *Side Effects Worksheet* on page 104 and report them to your doctors.

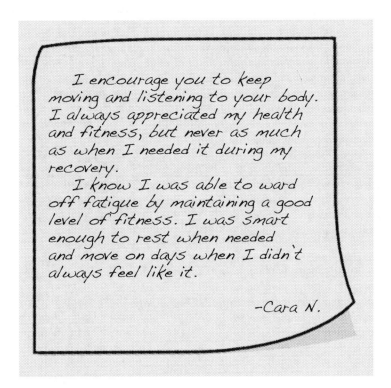

I encourage you to keep moving and listening to your body. I always appreciated my health and fitness, but never as much as when I needed it during my recovery.

I know I was able to ward off fatigue by maintaining a good level of fitness. I was smart enough to rest when needed and move on days when I didn't always feel like it.

—Cara N.

Questions for the Exercise Specialist

Is exercise recommended for me?   ❑ Yes   ❑ No

How will treatments affect me physically? _____

_____

_____

_____

_____

What can I do to lessen side effects? _____

_____

_____

_____

What types of fitness evaluations should I have prior to beginning exercise therapy?

❑ Body Fat Measurement   ❑ Aerobic Capacity Test   ❑ Muscular Endurance Test

Where can I have these test performed and by who? _____

_____

_____

What types of exercise can I do and how often? _____

_____

_____

What do I need to report immediately? _____

_____

_____

May I speak with other patients of yours?   ❑ Yes   ❑ No

Will the cost of the treatment be covered by my health insurance?   ❑ Yes   ❑ No

If not, are there financial assistance programs to help cover the costs?   ❑ Yes   ❑ No

Additional questions/comments: _____

_____

_____

_____

Exercise Log

Date	Activity	Time	Intensity (heart rate)	Comments/Thoughts/Reactions

Exercise Log

Notes

13

Complementary Therapy

Exploring Your Options

Athletes often use cross training (trying different activities outside of their main sport) to improve their performance. **Complementary therapies,** sometimes called **integrative therapies**, are a little like cross training since they are used in combination with conventional medical treatments.

> *Complementary therapy should not be confused with alternative medicines. Alternative medicines are forms of treatment used instead of conventional medical treatments and are not recommended.*

Complementary therapies can be very useful in managing your cancer and treatment-related symptoms. They can offer a sense of empowerment and control, helping improve your mental outlook, but they don't kill cancer. Any decisions about them should be made with your treatment team. Use the *Complementary Therapy Questions* on page 166 when talking about what you would like to try and why.

Types of Complementary Therapy

Complementary therapies are either passive (in which someone does something to you, such as a massage) or active (in which you are the one doing something, such as exercise). *(See Table 13.1)*

Table 13.1: Complementary Therapies	
Type	**Examples**
Natural therapy: A type of therapy that includes using herbal medicines, also known as botanicals. Many are sold over the counter as dietary supplements.	• Macrobiotic diet • Minerals • Soy • Vitamins
Mind-body therapy: This therapy focuses on the interactions between the mind and the body, with the intent to use the mind to affect physical functioning and promote health.	• Biofeedback • Guided imagery • Meditation • Prayer • Yoga
Energy therapy: These modalities are based on the idea that the human body has energy fields that can be stimulated through various techniques in order to promote wellness.	• Acupuncture • Alexander technique • Aromatherapy • Qi Gong • Reiki • Tai Chi
Manipulative and body-based practices: Focus primarily on manipulating the structures and systems of the body (including the bones and joints, soft tissues, circulatory and lymphatic systems) to promote healing and help control pain.	• Acupressure • Chiropractic • Massage therapy • Feldenkrais • Reflexology • Rolfing

Potential Side Effects

Talk with your healthcare team about complementary therapies you are using or considering in order to avoid harmful interactions with your standard medical treatments. Keep track of your therapies using the *Complementary Therapy Log* on page 167. Record any negative reactions on the *Side Effects Worksheet* on page 104.

> Two days after my treatments I would be slammed into bed for 3 to 4 days. I could hardly sip water, much less eat, due to nausea. The fatigue was debilitating; a short shower wore me out. I went to an acupuncturist at the cancer center where I was being treated with little expectation.
>
> The following day I had my chemotherapy and waited for the nausea and fatigue. By day four my husband kept looking at me and I just shrugged. The extreme symptoms were gone. I could eat, drink, and even take 45-minute morning walks.
>
> —Cindy S.

Complementary Therapy Questions

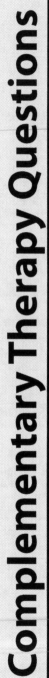

How do you feel about complementary therapies? _____

_____

Do you think complementary therapy would be good for me? ❑ Yes ❑ No

If so, which types of therapy would help me physically? _____

_____

Which types of therapy would help me emotionally? _____

_____

What's the best way to find a certified practitioner? _____

_____

I am currently using these therapies: _____

Should I stop them during and/or after my treatment? ❑ Yes ❑ No

Should I let you know before I start a complementary therapy? ❑ Yes ❑ No

Which therapies should I be sure to avoid? _____

Will complementary therapy interfere with my breast cancer treatment? ❑ Yes ❑ No

Are there potential dangers if I use complementary therapies? ❑ Yes ❑ No
If so, what are they? _____

Is there a clinical trial studying your recommended therapy? ❑ Yes ❑ No

Will the cost of the treatment be covered by my health insurance? ❑ Yes ❑ No

Additional questions/comments: _____

_____

_____

_____

_____

Complementary Therapy Log

Date	Activity	Comments/Thoughts/Reactions

Complementary Therapy Log

Notes

> *There will come a time when you believe everything is finished. That will be the beginning.*
>
> **- Louis L'Amour**

chapter 14

Mission Accomplished

Exploring Aftercare

You have just crossed the treatment finish line. Is it really over? Well, kind of. Your treatment is over but your aftercare is just beginning. Aftercare refers to your life after breast cancer treatment and the adjustments you will need to make. It begins the day your treatment ends and will last your entire lifetime. In many ways your life will resemble the life you had before cancer, but in other ways it will be different. Consider this your "new perspective."

Beginning Aftercare

When treatment ends, suddenly all the appointments, medical attention, and support you relied on seem to disappear, leaving you with an overwhelming sense of "Now what?" Once again, don't panic. It's time to formulate your post-treatment plan and set new goals. Some physical and emotional challenges may await you, but you will be able to handle them. Knowing what they may be is the first step.

Am I Cured?

At this time there is no definitive answer or test that can tell you if you are completely cancer free or cured. However, your chances of long-term survival can increase dramatically based on the type and stage of your cancer, your treatment choices, and your follow-up care. The good news is that statistics show an extremely high survival rate after the five-year mark for early-stage breast cancer patients. The longer you go without a recurrence, the less likely you are to experience one.

Fear of Recurrence

You may find yourself terrified every time you get a headache, cold, or bruise. You were never expecting to have breast cancer in the first place. In fact, you may have felt you were at the peak of your health when you were hit with the news. So how do you trust your body again?

Give it time. Reestablishing familiar routines, living a healthy lifestyle, joining support groups, and adhering to a strict follow-up schedule will all help you manage your fears.

> *I was fortunate enough to discover my breast cancer while performing a breast self-exam. What I now realize is that I wasn't even doing that thorough of a job. Don't be afraid to really explore your breast after treatments.*
>
> *Feel around using different angles and remember to check your lymph nodes. You do not need to be a hypochondriac, but you can't ignore your breasts either.*
>
> *—Cara N.*

Self-Examinations

It is true that once you have had breast cancer, you have an increased risk of getting cancer again. This is why it is extremely important to continue with self-examinations and regular medical exams after your treatment has ended. Perform breast and lymph node self-examinations every month, a few days after your menstrual period. If you no longer have periods, choose the same day each month for your exams, perhaps the first day of every month. Exams should be performed standing up and lying down. The American Cancer Society recommends the following steps for a breast self-exam. (*See Figure 14.1*)

Looking

Start with good lighting. Stand in front of a mirror naked from the waist up with your arms at your sides. Look for dimpling, puckering, or redness of the breast skin; discharge from the nipples; and changes in breast size or shape. Check for the same signs with your hands pressed tightly on your hips. Next, bend forward with your hands on your hips and check for any irregularities. Raise your arms high and turn to each side to check your breasts in profile. Look for any changes between the right and left breast. Remember it is common for one breast to be larger than the other, and for breasts to feel lumpy and uneven.

Feeling

Approaching your breasts from different positions helps you to feel and examine a wider area of tissue. The side-lying position lets you examine the outer half of the breast and stops your breast tissue from falling into the underarm area. A back-lying position allows you better access to the inner half of the breast. A standing position gives you better access to your lymph nodes. It's much easier to feel your breast tissue if you use a light lotion on your hands or soap if you're in the shower.

1. Place a folded towel or a pillow under your right shoulder while lying on your back with your knees bent. Put your right hand under or over your head.

2. With your left hand, keeping the fingers flat and together, gently feel your right breast without lifting your hand or changing the pressure.

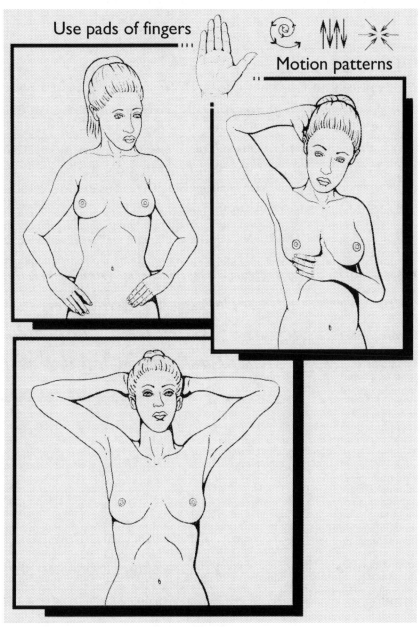

Figure 14.1

3. Use the flat part of your fingers (the pads) to examine your breast. Move your finger pads around the breast in a circular, line, or wedge pattern. Find the pattern that works best for you. Repeat the exam using three different pressures:

   - Light: barely move the top layer of skin
   - Medium: press halfway through the thickness of your breast
   - Deep: press to the base of the breast near the ribs

4. Make sure you examine the entire breast area from the middle of your armpit to the middle of your chest and all the way up to your collarbone.

5. Repeat steps one through three using a side-lying position, slightly rotating your bent knees to the opposite side of the breast you are examining.

6. Lower your right arm and perform the exam on the other breast, repeating steps one through four.

Standing Exam

While standing in front of a mirror be on the lookout for any unusual resistance, hardness, or lump beneath the nipples. Gently squeeze your nipples and look for any changes in appearance, discharge, or cracking. Next, examine the lymph nodes in each armpit, the surrounding areas under the arms and above the collarbones. Check the depressed areas near your neck above your collarbone by shrugging your shoulders and feeling along the area. Lymph nodes can be soft or hard and are shaped like peas. Sometimes lymph nodes are enlarged due to cancer. They can also become enlarged due to an infection.

It is extremely important—and your responsibility—to monitor your health between your scheduled visits. In fact, most recurrent breast cancer is suspected or detected by the patient between scheduled visits.

What to Report

Report any changes in your breasts, nipples, or lymph nodes. Call your doctor if you have any of the following symptoms:

- Lumps
- Swelling
- Skin irritation
- Dimpling

- Pain
- Nipple retraction (turning in) or discharge
- Redness of nipple or breast skin
- Scaly nipple or breast skin

Follow-Up Medical Exams

Don't toss out your appointment book just yet. Even though your treatments are over, you will still be in contact with your aftercare team often. They will want to see you at regularly scheduled intervals for at least the next five years. Spacing your visits throughout the year will ensure you are being seen by someone on your aftercare team every ten to twelve weeks.

What to Report

If you start to experience any of the following symptoms, contact a member of your aftercare team so you can be evaluated as soon as possible.

- Any changes in the remaining breast(s) and chest area

- New lumps in the breast(s), chest wall, armpit, or neck

- Unusual chest pain, backaches, or bone pain

- Loss of appetite or weight changes, especially weight loss

- Changes in menstrual periods or unusual vaginal bleeding

- Dizziness, rapid vision changes, or headaches

- Coughing that does not go away, hoarseness, or shortness of breath

- Skin rashes or chronic swelling

- Unusual digestive tract problems that won't go away

Your follow-up guidelines will be established by your aftercare treatment team. Below are some typical scheduling recommendations:

- **Physical exam**—Recommended for all patients every four to six months for five years, then every twelve months.

- **Mammogram**—For patients treated with lumpectomy and radiation: every six months after radiation therapy ends, then every six to twelve months. For patients with mastectomy: every twelve months.

- **Pelvic exam/pap smear**—For women who have not had their uterus removed: every twelve months.

- **Bone health exams**—For all patients every twelve months.

Refer to your *Questions for the Aftercare Team Worksheet* on page 176 when speaking with your doctors during your follow-up appointments.

Riding the Emotional Roller Coaster

It's very common for your emotions to be all over the place. You have been through a lot. Luckily, you are not alone and there is always someone to turn to. More than two million people have faced the breast cancer battle and won. Take advantage of support groups and programs and always discuss your feelings and concerns with your aftercare team.

Establish a Healthy Lifestyle

Diet

There is no "magic" cancer diet that has been proven to prevent recurrence. But there is strong evidence that maintaining a healthy body weight lowers the chance of recurrence. Since fat can encourage estrogen production, which in turn can trigger breast cancer cell growth, it is extremely important to maintain a healthy body weight. Ask your doctor what your ideal weight is. The following guidelines can help you stay on track:

- Try to eat at least five servings of fruits and vegetables daily.

- Choose whole grain foods more often.

- Add flax seed to your diet.

- Make olive oil your primary fat.

- Get enough vitamin D and calcium every day.

- Limit red meat, processed meat, and sugar.

- Drink little to no alcohol. There is increasing evidence that alcohol consumption increases breast cancer risk.

> Stay positive. Keep living a full life. You often hear the phrase "There is no cure for cancer." I chose not to think that way. Life right now is good and I hope to have many more such years.
> I think we can overcome so much by opening our eyes to the gifts and happiness we have rather than dwelling on those that we no longer have. Life itself is a miracle. Enjoy it.
>
> –Joyce B.

Exercise

Exercise was important before you had cancer and is even more so now. Consider exercise as a primary prescription in your aftercare. Why is it so darn important? Here's what exercising regularly does for you:

- Stimulates your body's ability to fight off and destroy infections and disease.

- Lowers body fat mass, reducing your risk of recurrence.

- Aids in managing menopausal symptoms.

- Increases your endorphins, substances that reduce pain and promote a feeling of well-being.

- Increases bone density, which can be affected by your cancer treatment.

- Lowers your risk factors for cardiovascular disease, diabetes, and other cancers.

Before starting any new exercise program, be sure to consult with your aftercare team. Start slowly and report any issues or concerns you have. If you can, work with a certified cancer specialist from the American College of Sports Medicine or the Cancer Exercise Training Institute. Work your way up to the following:

- Thirty minutes of moderately intense cardiovascular exercise five days a week. "Moderate intensity" means working hard enough to raise your heart rate and break a sweat, yet still being able to carry on a conversation.

- Eight to ten strength-training exercises in eight to twleve repetitions twice a week. Be sure to speak with your surgeon regarding concerns about lymphedema.

Reevaluating Your Priorities

Cancer is a life-changing event. Even though you have resumed your normal activities and fallen into old patterns, your view of life may never be the same. In fact, it may be better than ever. During treatment it is very common to reflect on your life choices. During aftercare it is more common to act on them.

Paying It Forward

During your treatment, you most likely encountered people who were tremendously helpful to you with no expectations in return. Now take the opportunity to **pay it forward**. Instead of "paying back" those helpful people, you can "pay it forward" by doing a good deed for someone else.

You might decide to pay it forward by donating your time or resources to breast cancer research. It could be as simple an act as donating magazines to your doctor's waiting room or driving another patient to an appointment. Whatever you feel comfortable doing is the right action for you. Paying it forward not only helps others, it benefits your immune system as well, and who couldn't use that?

Moving Forward

Will you ever be able to forget about breast cancer? No. However, you will be able to move beyond it. There was life before your cancer and there is a wonderful life awaiting you after your treatment. Facing your fears, talking about all that you have been through, and setting new goals will help keep you moving forward.

Questions for the Aftercare Team

Is my cancer gone?   ❑ Yes   ❑ No

What is my prognosis? _____
_____

What are my chances of recurrence? _____

How will you monitor me? _____

Who should I see and how often? _____
_____

What short-term side-effects might I have? _____
_____

What long-term side effects might I have? _____
_____

Who can I talk to about my feelings? _____

What should I report immediately? _____
_____

What are my chances of getting lypmhedema? _____

What signs should I look out for? _____
_____
_____

What should I eat? _____
_____

How often should I exercise? _____
_____

What should I use for birth control? _____

What if I want children? _____
_____

Additional questions/comments: _____
_____
_____
_____
_____

Treatment Summary

Diagnosis Information

Date of Diagnosis: _____/_____/_____

Age at Diagnosis: _____

Family History: ❑ None ❑ 1st Degree Relative ❑ 2nd Degree Relative

Previous Breast Cancer: ❑ No ❑ Yes : _____/_____/_____

Date of Tissue Diagnosis: _____

Hormonal Status at Time of Diagnosis: ❑ Pre-Menopausal ❑ Post-Menopausal

Date of last period: _____/_____/_____

Pathology Findings

Date of Biopsy: ___/___/___	Pathologist:
Type of Cancer:	Tumor Size:
# of Nodes removed:	# of Nodes positive:
Breast: ❑ Right ❑ Left ❑ Bilateral	Surgical Margins Clear: ❑ Yes ❑ No

Stage: ❑ 0 ❑ I ❑ 2A ❑ 2B ❑ 3A ❑ 3B ❑ 3C ❑ 4

ER Status: ❑ Positive ❑ Negative PR Status: ❑ Positive ❑ Negative

HER-2/neu Status: ❑ Positive ❑ Negative

Surgical Treatment

Date: _____/_____/_____

Breast Surgeon: _____ Phone: _____

Hospital: _____

Type: ❑ Lumpectomy ❑ Mastectomy ❑ Mastectomy & Immediate Reconstructive
      ❑ Axillary Dissection ❑ Sentinel Node Biopsy

Reconstructive Surgeon: _____ Phone: _____

Hospital: _____

Type of Reconstructive Surgery: _____

Complications or comments: _____

_____

Treatment Summary

Treatment Summary

Radiation Treatment

Radiation Oncologist:_____ Phone: _____

Type: ❑ Internal   ❑ External   ❑ Whole Breast   ❑ Partial Breast

❑ Local (breast)   ❑ Regional (nodes)

Any complications: _____

Location	Area	Type	Prescribed Dose	Fraction Number	Elapsed Days	Treatment From	To

Hormonal & Biological Treatment Summary

Medical Oncologist: _____ Phone: _____

Type of Treatment: ❑ None

❑ Trastuzumab (Herceptin)   from: ____/____/____   to: ____/____/____

❑ Tamoxifen   from: ____/____/____   to: ____/____/____

❑ Aromatase Inhibitor   from: ____/____/____   to: ____/____/____

❑ Other: _____   from: ____/____/____   to: ____/____/____

❑ Other: _____   from: ____/____/____   to: ____/____/____

Administered: ❑ by Pill   ❑ by IV   ❑ Surgically

Complications or comments: _____

_____

Genetic Testing

Date of Test: ____/____/____

Name of Genetic Counselor: _____ Phone: _____

Name & Address of Institution: _____

My Results: BRCA 1:   ❑ Negative   ❑ Positive   BRCA2:   ❑ Negative   ❑ Positive

Who interpreted the results: _____

Treatment Summary

Chemotherapy

Medical Oncologist: _____ Phone: _____

Pre-Treatment Weight _____ lb/kg   Post-Treatment Weight _____ lb/kg

Date of last menstrual period pre treatment: _____/_____/_____

Date of last menstrual period post treatment: _____/_____/_____

Name of Regime: _____

Name of Clinical Trial: _____

Contact Name: _____ Phone: _____

Start Date: _____/_____/_____   End Date _____/_____/_____

Drug Name	Route	Dose	Schedule	Dose reduction needed	Number of cycles
				❑ Yes ___% ❑ No	
				❑ Yes ___% ❑ No	
				❑ Yes ___% ❑ No	
				❑ Yes ___% ❑ No	
				❑ Yes ___% ❑ No	
				❑ Yes ___% ❑ No	

Side Effects:

- ❑ Hair loss
- ❑ Nausea/Vomiting
- ❑ Neuropathy
- ❑ Fatigue
- ❑ Low blood count
- ❑ Menopause

Serious toxicities during treatment:_____

Additional drugs administered: _____

Allergic events: _____

Complications or comments: _____

_____

_____

Notes

> *What lies behind us, and what lies before us, are tiny matters compared to what lies within us.*
>
> *- Ralph Waldo Emerson*

chapter 15

Facing a Recurrence

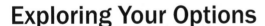

Exploring Your Options

Luckily, most people will never experience a recurrence (a cancer that has come back). However, if breast cancer does come back it is most likely to occur in the first two to five years after initial treatment. Continue monthly breast self-exams and keep your scheduled follow-up appointments. If you suspect a recurrence, meet with your treatment team immediately. Use the *Recurrence Questions Worksheet* on page 184 along with the *Recurrence Treatment Options Worksheet* on page 185 to help guide you in formulating your new treatment plan.

What should you look out for?

According to WebMD.com, some indicators put you at a higher risk for recurrence based on your initial breast cancer. Your risk can increase if you had the following indicators:

- Lymph node involvement

- Lymphatic system or blood vessel involvement

- Large tumor size

- ER-negative hormone receptors

- Poorly differentiated cells

- High nuclear grade

- HER-2/neu positive

Any changes in your breasts should be reported immediately. Signs and symptoms to look out for include:

• A lump or thickening	• Pain
• Swelling	• Skin irritation
• Change in breast appearance	• Redness of nipple or breast skin
• Dimpling	• Scaly nipple or breast skin
• Nipple retraction (turning in)	• Nipple discharge

Types of Recurrence

Recurrences usually occur because the original treatment didn't destroy all of the cancer cells. This can happen when cancer cells have remained undetected, have been dormant, or are resistant to treatment. The type of treatment and predicted outcomes for breast cancer recurrences will depend on both your initial treatment and the type of recurrence you have. There are four different types of breast cancer recurrence:

1. Local recurrence refers to cancer that comes back in the same area or near the location of the original cancer. Local recurrences occur:

   - After breast-conserving surgery: This type of local recurrence usually shows up three to five years later in the original site of breast conservation surgery due to cancer cells that survived the first treatment.

   - After mastectomy: This type of local recurrence can occur under the skin and fat in the chest wall or near the mastectomy scar. Most of these recurrences appear within the first five years following the mastectomy.

2. Regional recurrence refers to cancer that has returned to lymph nodes.

   - Axillary recurrence occurs in the armpit (axillary) region. This type of recurrence is very rare.

   - Supraclavical recurrence occurs in the lymph nodes located above the collarbone.

3. New primary refers to a new cancer that generally happens many years later and in an entirely different area of the breast. Although it is referred to as a recurrence, a new primary tumor should be treated as a completely new cancer, just as a second cancer in the opposite breast would be treated.

4. Distant recurrence or metastatic disease refers to cancer that has spread to other areas of the body, usually the lungs, bones, or liver.

Starting Over

Don't beat yourself up questioning all of your previous treatment decisions and wondering if you made the right choices. Rest assured that you made the best treatment choices that were available to you at the time and you can do it again. You may have new goals now, but you have learned how to break them down into manageable steps.

Sometimes facing a recurrence is not as scary as facing cancer the first time, because you have already taken the time to do research, ask questions, and explore treatment options. You can maintain a sense of control while treating your recurrent cancer using the same approach and tools that you did before.

It was a shock to be dealing with breast cancer again, and scary. The good news was that I went in for a routine mammogram, was asked if I could wait for an ultrasound (immediately I knew something was up), and only waited an hour for the ultrasound—in other words, no waiting at least a week for each next step.

At the end of the ultrasound, the radiologist squeezed my hand and said, "Look at it this way; you've beaten it before so you can beat it again." This was not good news, but having such a fast diagnosis was very helpful psychologically.

—Holly H.

Recurrence Questions

Recurrence Questions

What type of recurrence do I have? _____

What are my treatment options? *(See Recurrence Treatment Options on page 185).* _____
_____
_____

How often have you seen this type of recurrence after my first cancer and treatments?
_____
_____

Does this change anything for my family members?   ❑ Yes   ❑ No
If yes, what? _____
_____
_____

Is there another specialist I should see?   ❑ Yes   ❑ No
If yes, who? _____

What is my prognosis? _____

What support is available to me? _____
_____
_____

Additional questions/comments: _____
_____
_____
_____
_____
_____
_____
_____
_____
_____

Recurrence Treatment Options

List the advantages and disadvantages of each option you are a candidate for.

Opinion given by: _____

Option: _____

Treatment length: _____ Odds of Cure: _____

Risks: _____

_____

_____

_____

Side effects: _____

_____

_____

_____

_____

Other factors: _____

_____

_____

_____

Option: _____

Treatment length: _____ Odds of Cure: _____

Risks: _____

_____

_____

_____

Side effects: _____

_____

_____

_____

_____

Other factors: _____

_____

_____

_____

Notes

Part III
Additional Resources

It's easy to get lost, waylaid, or just plain confused with all the information on the Internet. The following tips can help you stay on track when searching the information highway:

- Search sites that end in .edu or .org.

- Know who is answering your questions. Are they experts, fellow cancer patients, or companies trying to sell you something?

- Check the date of website postings to make sure the information is current.

- Use these guidelines for books, magazines, and journal articles as well.

As you gather more information, please keep in mind that educational resources are designed to complement sound medical advice, never replace it.

Internet Resources

General Resources

About.Com
www.breastcancer.about.com

Adjuvant Online
www.adjuvantonline.com

African American Breast Cancer Alliance, Inc. (AABCA)
www.aabcainc.org

American Cancer Society (ACS)
www.cancer.org
1-800-ACS-2345 (1-800-227-2345)

Beyond the Shock
www.breastcancer.net

BreastCancer.org
www.breastcancer.org

Breast Cancer Network of Strength
www.networkofstrength.org
24-hour hotline (English): 1-800-221-2141
(Spanish): 1-800-986-9505

Dr. Susan Love's Research Foundation
www.dslrf.org

eMedicineHealth
www.emedicinehealth.com/breast

I'm Too Young For This! Cancer Foundation
www.stupidcancer.com

Inflammatory Breast Cancer Association
www.ibchelp.org

International Cancer Alliance for Research and Education
www.icare.org

MEDLINEplus: Breast Cancer
www.nlm.nih.gov

National Cancer Institute (NCI)
www.nci.nih.gov
1-800-4-CANCER (1-800-422-6237)

National Alliance of Breast Cancer Organizations (NABCO)
www.nabco.org

National Breast Cancer Coalition
www.stopbreastcancer.org
1-800-622-2838

National Breast Cancer Foundation
www.nationalbreastcancer.org

National Cancer Institute (NCI)
www.nci.nih.gov
1-800-4-CANCER (1-800-422-6237)

National Comprehensive Cancer Network (NCCN)
www.nccn.com

Navigating Cancer
www.navigatingcancer.com

Susan G. Komen for the Cure
www.komen.org
1-877-465-6636

Y-ME National Breast Cancer Organization
www.y-me.org

WebMD Breast Cancer Health Center
www.webmd.com/cancer

The Young Survival Coalition
www.youngsurvival.org

Aftercare

Journey Forward
www.journeyforward.org

Life After Cancer Care
www.mdanderson.org/survivorship

Livestrong Care Plan
www.livestrongcareplan.org.

National Coalition for Cancer Survivorship
www.canceradvocacy.org
1-877-622-7937

Reach to Recovery: The American Cancer Society (ACS)
www.cancer.org/Treatment/
SupportProgramsServices/reach-to-recovery
1-800-ACS-2345 (1-800-227-2345)

Appearance

Facing the Mirror
www.facingthemirror.org

Look Good, Feel Better
www.lookgoodfeelbetter.org
1-800-395-LOOK (1-800-395-5665)

Tender Loving Care—American Cancer Society
www.tlcdirect.org

Breast Surgeons

American College of Surgeons
www.facs.org

American Society of Breast Surgeons
www.breastsurgeons.org

American Society of Plastic and Reconstructive Surgeons
www.plasticsurgery.org

U.S. Food and Drug Administration
www.fda.gov

Caregiving

Care Calendar
www.carecalendar.org

CancerCare
www.cancercare.org
1-800-813-4673

Cancer Support Community
www.thewellnesscommunity.org/mm/Caring/
Caregiver-Support

Family Caregiver Alliance (FCA)/ National Center on Caregiving
www.caregiver.org

Clinical Trials

BreastcancerTrials.org
www.BreastCancerTrials.org

Cancer.gov: Breast Cancer Clinical Trials
www.cancer.gov/clinicaltrials

CancerConsultants.com
www.cancerconsultants.com

Clinical Trials
www.ClinicalTrials.gov
1-800-4-CANCER

Coalition of National Cancer Cooperative Groups
www.cancertrialshelp.org/trialcheck

National Institute of Health's MedlinePlus
www.nlm.nih.gov/medlineplus

Complementary Therapy

American Association of Acupuncture and Oriental Medicine
www.aaaomonline.org

American Art Therapy Association Inc.
www.arttherapy.org

American Massage Therapy Association
www.amtamassage.org

American Music Therapy Association
www.musictherapy.org

Association for Applied Psychophysiology and Biofeedback
www.aapb.org

Cancer Support Community (The)
www.cancersupportcommunity.org

National Center for Complementary and Alternative Medicine (NCCAM)
www.nccam.nih.gov
1-888-644-6226

National Center for Homeopathy
www.homeopathic.org

National Cancer Institute's Office of Cancer Complementary and Alternative Medicine (OCCAM)
www.cancer.gov/cam
1-800-4-CANCER (1-800-422-6237)

Society of Integrative Oncology
www.integrativeonc.org

Exercise

American College of Sports Medicine
www.acsm.org
1-800-877-1600

Cancer Exercise Training Institute
www.thecancerspecialist.com/specialist.aspx

National Center for Complementary and Alternative Medicine (NCCAM)
www.nccam.nih.gov
1-888-644-6226

Family History

Facing Our Risk of Cancer Empowered (FORCE)
www.facingourrisk.org

National Human Genome Research Institute
www.genome.gov/11510372

National Society of Genetic Counselors (NSGC)
www.NSCG.org

NorthShore University HealthSystems
www.northshore.org/mygenerations

Family Support

Cancer Support Community
www.gildasclub.org

Kids Konnected
www.kidskonnected.org
1-800-899-2866

Mothers Supporting Daughters With Breast Cancer (MSDBC)
www.motherdaughters.org

National Students of AMF (Ailing Mothers & Fathers) Support Network
www.studentsofamf.org

Fertility

Fertile HOPE
www.fertilehope.org

My Oncofertility
www.myoncofertility.org

Lymphedema

Lymphatic Research Foundation
www.lymphaticresearch.org

National Lymphedema Network
www.lymphnet.org

Male Breast Cancer

The American Cancer Society (ACS): Male Breast Cancer Resource Center
www.cancer.org/cancer/breastcancerinmen

Medical Oncology & Chemotherapy

Adjuvant! Online
www.adjuvantonline.com

American Society of Clinical Oncology (ACSO)
www.cancer.net
1-888-282-2552

National Institute of Health's MedlinePlus
www.nlm.nih.gov/medlineplus

Triple Negative Breast Cancer Foundation
www.tnbcfoundation.org

Nutrition

American Botanical Council
abc.herbalgram.org
1-800-373-7105

American Cancer Society
www.cancer.org
1-800-227-2345

American Dietetic Association
www.eatright.org
1-800-877-1600

BreastCancer.org
www.breastcancer.org

National Cancer Institute (NCI) Eating Hints
www.cancer.gov/cancerinfo/eatinghints
1-800-4-CANCER (1-800-422-6237)

National Center for Complementary and Alternative Medicine (NCCAM)
www.nccam.nih.gov
1-888-644-6226

Office of Dietary Supplements
www.ods.od.nih.gov
1-301-435-2920

Patient Travel

Air Charity
www.aircharitynetwork.org

Angel Flight
www.angelflight.com

Hope Lodge: American Cancer Society
www.cancer.org/Treatment/
SupportProgramsServices/HopeLodge/index

Joe's House
www.joeshouse.org

National Association of Hospital Hospitality Houses
www.nahhh.org

Practical Matters

Cancer and Careers
www.cancerandcareers.org

Cancer Legal Resource Center (CLRC)
www.lls.edu/academics/candp/clrc.html

Cancer Supportive Care
www.cancersupportivecare.com/drug_assistance.
html

Health Insurance Association of America (HIAA)
www.ahip.org/content/default.aspx?bc=41

Medicaid
www.cms.gov/home/medicaid.asp

Patient Advocate Foundation
www.patientadvocate.org
1-800-532-5274

National Foundation for Credit Counseling (NFCC)
www.nfcc.org

National Coalition for Cancer Survivorship (NCCS)
www.canceradvocacy.org
1-301-650-9127

National Hospice Organization (NHPO)
www.nhpo.org

National Partnership for Women & Families
www.nationalpartnership.org

Needy Meds
www.needymeds.com

Partnership for Prescription Assistance
www.pparx.org

Pharmaceutical Research and Manufacturers of America (PhRMA)
www.phrma.org

Social Security
www.social-security-disability-claims.org

US Department of Health and Human Services: Agency for Healthcare Research and Quality
www.ahrq.gov/consumer

US Department of Health and Human Services: Medicare
www.medicare.gov
1-800-MEDICARE (1-800-633-4227)

US Department of Veterans Affairs
www.va.gov
1-800-827-1000

Pregnancy

Hope for Two: Pregnant with Cancer Network
www.hopefortwo.org
1-800-743-4471

The National Comprehensive Cancer Network (NCCN)
www.nccn.com

Pregnant with Cancer Network
www.pregnantwithcancer.org
1-800-743-4471

Prostheses

The American Cancer Society (ACS)
www.cancer.org/Cancer/BreastCancer/
DetailedGuide/breast-cancer-after-body-image
1-800-ACS-2345 (1-800-227-2345)

Breast Cancer Network of Strength
www.networkofstrength.org
24-hour Hotline (English): 1-800-221-2141
(Spanish): 1-800-986-9505

Lucy's International Breast Forms
www.lucys.net
1-866-264-9500

Radiation

American College of Radiology (ACR)
www.acr.org

American Society for Radiation Oncology (ASTRO)
www.astro.org
1-800-962-7876

Recurrence

AdvancedBC.org
www.advancedbc.org

Metastatic Breast Cancer Network (MBCN)
www.mbcnetwork.org

Support and Advocacy Groups

American Cancer Society (ACS)
www.cancer.org
1-800-ACS-2345 (1-800-227-2345)

Association of Cancer Online Resources
www.ACOR.org

CancerCare
www.cancercare.org
1-800-813-HOPE (1-800-813-4673)

Cancer Hope Network
www.cancerhope.org
1-800-552-4366

Cleaning for a Reason (free household support)
www.cleaningforareason.org
1-877-337-3348

Facing Our Rirsk of Cancer Empowered (FORCE)
www.facingourrisk.org

Imerman Angels
www.imermansngels.org
1-877-274-5529

Journey Through Cancer
www.journeythroughcancer.org

KidsHealth for Kids
http://kidshealth.org/kid/grownup/conditions/
breast_cancer.html

Kids Konnected
www.kidskonnected.org
1-800-899-2866

Livestrong
www.livestrong.org
1-866-676-7250

Men Against Breast Cancer
www.menagainstbreastcancer.org/about/

**National Asian Women's Health Organization
(NAWHO)**
www.nawho.org

National Coalition for Cancer Survivorship
www.canceradvocacy.org
1-877-622-7937

Patient Advocate Foundation (PFA)
www.patientadvocate.org
1-800-532-5274

**People Living with Cancer (Buddy Support
Network)**
www.plwc.org.za

Right Action For Women
www.rightactionforwomen.org

Sisters Network Inc.
www.sistersnetworkinc.org
1-866-781-1808

Susan G. Komen for the Cure
www.komen.org
1-800-IM-AWARE (1-800-462-9273)

The Young Survival Coalition
www.youngsurvival.org

Understanding Lab & Imaging Tests

Labs Tests Online
www.labtestsonline.org/understanding/

Oncotype DX
www.oncotypedx.com

Young Adults

I'm Too Young For This! Cancer Foundation
www.stupidcancer.com

Planet Cancer
www.planetcancer.org

The Young Survival Coalition
www.youngsurvival.org

Glossary

A

Adjuvant therapy: Treatment that is added to improve the effectiveness of surgical therapy.

Aftercare: Your life after breast cancer treatment and the adjustments you will need to make.

Alkylators: Drugs that interfere with the cell's DNA and inhibit cancer cell growth.

Anthracyclines: Drugs that change the structure of cellular DNA.

Antimetabolites: Drugs that interfere with cancer cell division needed to make new DNA.

Antimitotic: Drugs that prevent cancer cells from dividing.

Areola: The dark area of skin around the nipple.

Aromatase inhibitors: Drugs which prevent fat, muscle cells, and the adrenal glands from producing estrogen in post-menopausal women. They stop an enzyme called aromatase from turning other hormones into estrogen.

Autologous: Taken from your own tissues, cells or DNA.

Axilla: Armpit

Axillary lymph node: Lymph nodes found in the armpit area.

Axillary lymph node dissection: Surgical removal of lymph nodes found in the armpit region.

B

Benign tumor: An abnormal growth that is not cancer, is self-limited and does not invade or metastasize.

Biological therapy: Also called targeted therapy. Treatment used to stimulate or restore the ability of the immune system to fight cancer, infections, and other diseases. Agents used in biological therapy include monoclonal antibodies, growth factors, and vaccines. They take advantage of your body's own immune system to act on cancer cells with little harm to your healthy cells, for example Herceptin.

Biopsy: Removal of a small piece of your tissue or tumor to examine your cells.

Blood count: Your blood may be drawn and examined to evaluate your red blood cells (RBC), white blood cells (WBC), your platelets, electrolytes and hemoglobin, among other factors.

Bone marrow: The soft inner part of large bones that produces blood cells. Chemotherapy affects the bone marrow, resulting in a temporary decrease in the number of cells in the blood.

Bone scan: This procedure involves injecting a small amount of a radioactive substance into your bloodstream in order to see if cancer has spread to your bones.

Brachytherapy: Radiation that comes from a radioactive material placed in the body near cancer cells.

BRCA1 and BRCA2: Both are genes that are associated with the development of breast, ovarian and prostate cancers when inherited in a defective state.

Breast cancer: A mass of breast cells that is abnormal with uncontrolled growth.

Breast conservation surgery: Surgery which removes the tumor and varying degrees of the remaining breast tissue.

Breast implant: A silicone- or saline-filled sac inserted into the body to restore the shape of the breast.

Breast reconstruction: A type of surgery that uses either your own tissue or artificial material to rebuild a natural-looking breast.

Breast self-exam (BSE): A procedure to examine the breasts thoroughly once a month to detect any changes or suspicious lumps.

C

Cancer cell: A cell that divides and reproduces abnormally with uncontrolled growth. This cell can break away and travel to other parts of the body and set up at another site.

Capable companion: Someone who can be relied on to be a second set of eyes and ears throughout the treatment process.

Carcinoma: Cancer that starts in the skin or in the lining of the tissues that cover internal organs.

Caregiver: A person who provides physical, emotional, spiritual, or financial support to a patient.

CAT scan or CT scan: An x-ray view of the body in sections.

Cell: The basic structural unit of all life.

Cell differentiation: How much the tumor cells resemble the original (normal) cell.

Cellulitis: Infection of the soft tissues.

Chemotherapy: A treatment option that uses chemicals (drugs) to kill or disable cancer cells that are growing and dividing in your body.

Clavicle: The collarbone.

Clinical trials: A type of research that tests how well new medical approaches work.

Comedo: A non-invasive type of ductal cancer that tends to be slow-growing.

Complementary therapies: Also called integrative therapies, as they are integrated, or used in combination with conventional medical treatments.

Complete axillary dissection: When all levels of axillary nodes are removed.

Complete blood count (CBC): A laboratory test to determine the number of red blood cells, white blood cells, platelets, hemoglobin and other components of a blood sample.

Computerized tomography scans: Commonly called CT or CAT scans. These specialized x-ray studies indicate cancer or metastasis.

Consent form: A form explaining the procedure you will undergo, including any emergency procedures that may take place.

Core needle biopsy: Type of needle biopsy where a small core of tissue is removed from a lump without surgery.

Cribiform: A non-invasive type of ductal cancer that tends to be fast-growing.

Cytotoxic: Causing the death of cells. The term usually refers to drugs used in chemotherapy.

D

Diagnosis: The process of identifying a disease by its characteristic signs, symptoms and laboratory findings.

Differentiated: The similarity between a normal cell and the cancer cell; defines what degree of change has occurred. Cancer cells that are well-differentiated are close to the original cell and usually less aggressive. Poorly differentiated cells have changed more and are more aggressive.

Distant recurrence or metastatic disease: Refers to cancer that has spread to other areas of the body, usually the lungs, bone, or liver.

DNA (deoxyribonucleic acid): The molecules inside cells that carry genetic information.

DNA microarray analysis: A way of analyzing the many mutations in many tumors at the same time.

Dose dense: Chemotherapy in which the interval between two courses is shortened while the dose of each course may be increased, decreased or made equivalent to a standard dose so that the dose per unit of time is higher.

Drain bulbs: Bulbs that are designed to collect fluids that can accumulate post surgery.

Ductal carcinoma in situ (DCIS): A noninvasive form of cancer found in the lining of the breast duct.

Ducts: Tiny tubes that carry the milk from the lobules to the nipple.

E

Estrogen: Female sex hormone produced primarily by the ovaries that aids in developing female sex organs as well as regulating monthly menstrual cycles.

Estrogen receptor: Protein found on some cells to which estrogen molecules will attach. If a tumor is positive for estrogen receptors, it is sensitive to hormones.

Excisional biopsy: A procedure where a lump or suspicious tissue is surgically removed by cutting the skin and removing the tissue sample.

External-beam radiation therapy: Radiation that comes from a machine outside the body.

F

Fine needle aspiration: The removal of cells or fluid from tissues with a thin needle for microscopic examination.

FISH (Fluorescence In Situ Hybridization) test: A test that shows whether there are too many copies of the HER-2/neu gene in the cancer cells.

Flow cytometry: Test that measures DNA content in tumors.

Free-flap surgery: A surgery which involves removing muscle, skin and fat from your donor site, but does not leave the blood vessels attached during the transfer to the breast area. Instead, the removed tissue is placed directly into an opening in the chest area where the surgeon carefully reattaches the cut blood vessels to the new blood vessels under the armpit or in the chest wall.

Frozen shoulder: Stiffness or severe limitation of movement of the shoulder, due to scarring.

G

Gene microarray technology: This test uses a technique called gene chip technology to analyze all the genetic material in a cell.

Genetic testing: A test that analyzes DNA to look for a genetic mutation that may indicate an increased risk for developing a specific disease or disorder.

Genome: All of the chromosomes that together form the genetic map.

H

Hematoma: Collection of blood in the tissues. Hematomas may occur in the breast after surgery.

Her-2/neu: An oncogene that, when overexpressed, leads to more cell growth.

Hormone: Chemical substance produced by glands in the body which enters the bloodstream and causes effects in other tissues.

Hormonal therapy: A treatment given to block the body's naturally occurring estrogen and prevent the cancer from growing.

Hormone receptors: Hormone receptors are molecules, which are located on the surface of cells. These receptors recognize hormones circulating in your blood stream.

Hot flashes: Sudden, brief sensation of increased warmth and swelling associated with menopause.

I

IHC (ImunnoHistoChemistry) test: A test that shows whether there is too much of the HER-2/neu receptor protein in the cancer cells.

Immune system: Complex system that defends the body against infections and other diseases.

Immunology: The study of the body's ability to fight a disease.

Implants: A rubberlike silicone shell (sac) that is filled with saline or silicone gel and designed to recreate a breast following a mastectomy.

Incisional biopsy: A procedure where a portion of a lump or suspicious tissue is removed for diagnosis.

Inflammation: Reaction of tissue to various conditions that may result in pain, redness or warmth of tissues in the area.

Informed consent: Process in which the patient is fully informed of all risks and complications of a planned procedure and agrees to proceed.

In situ: In the site of. In regard to cancer, in situ refers to tumors that haven't grown beyond their site of origin and invaded neighboring tissue.

Internal radiation therapy: Radiation that comes from a radioactive material placed in the body near cancer cells.

Interstitial brachytherapy: Partial breast irradiation through tubes loaded with radioactive seeds.

Intracavitary brachytherapy: Partial breast irradiation through a balloon filling the biopsy cavity.

Intraductal: Within the duct. Intraductal can describe a benign or malignant process.

Intraductal papilloma: Benign tumor that projects like a finger from the lining of the duct.

Intramuscular (I.M.): Into a muscle.

Intraoperative radiation therapy (IORT): Irradiation applied in the operating room to the bed of the tumor.

Intravenous (I.V.): Into or within a vein.

Invasive cancer: Cancer that is capable of growing beyond its site of origin and invading neighboring tissue; also called infiltrating cancer.

Invasive ductal carcinoma (IDC): Cancer cells form in the lining of the milk duct, break free from the duct wall and invade the surrounding breast tissue.

Invasive lobular carcinoma (ILC): ILC starts in the milk producing lobule and invades the surrounding breast tissue.

Inverted nipple: A nipple that is turned inward.

L

Lactation: Production of milk from the breast.

Linear accelerator: A machine that produces high-energy x-ray beams to destroy cancer cells.

Lobular: Pertaining to the lobules of the breast.

Lobules: Milk-producing glands of the breast.

Localized cancer: A cancer still confined to its site of origin.

Local recurrence: Cancer that comes back in the same area or near where the original cancer was.

Local treatment of cancer: Treatment of the tumor only.

Lump: Any kind of abnormal mass in the breast or elsewhere in the body.

Lumpectomy: Surgery to remove lump with a small amount of normal tissue around it.

Lymph: A clear fluid circulating throughout the body in the lymphatic system that contains white blood cells and antibodies.

Lymphatic vessels: Vessels that carry lymphatic fluid to and from lymph nodes.

Lymphedema: This swelling of the arm can follow surgery to the lymph nodes under the arm. It can cause painful swelling in the hand or arm of the surgical side due to lymph fluid build-up.

Lymph nodes: Are a part of the lymphatic system and are glands that act as filters to stop bacteria and cellular waste from entering the blood stream. Lymph nodes can be a location of cancer spread.

M

Magnetic resonance imaging (MRI): A magnet scan; a form of x-ray using magnets instead of radiation. MRI gives a more clearly defined picture of fatty tissue than does an x-ray.

Malignant: Cancerous.

Malignant tumor: A group of cancer cells that may grow into (invade) surrounding tissues or spread (metastasize) to distant areas of the body.

Mammary glands: The breast glands that produce and carry milk by way of the mammary ducts to the nipples during pregnancy and breastfeeding.

Mammogram: An x-ray of the breast.

Margins: The area of tissue surrounding a tumor when it is removed by surgery.

Mastectomy: Surgical removal of the breast and some of the surrounding tissue.

Medical oncologist: A doctor who specializes in a wide variety of cancer treatments including chemical, hormonal, and biological therapies.

Menopause: The time in a woman's life when the menstrual cycle ends and the ovaries stop producing hormones.

Metastasis: The spread of cancer from one body part to another, usually through the blood stream.

Micrometastasis: Small numbers of cancer cells (microscopic) that have spread from the primary tumor and are too few to be detected on a diagnostic or screening test.

Mitosis: Cell division.

Modified radical mastectomy: Surgery for breast cancer in which all of the breast tissue, the nipple and areola, the lining of the pectoral muscle, and the axillary (underarm) lymph nodes are removed.

Monoclonal antibody: A laboratory designed protein.

Multicentric: More than one tumor or place of growth in the breast. These growths are likely to be located in different quadrants of the breast.

Multifocal: More than one tumor, all of which have arisen from the original tumor. These tumors are likely to be located in the same quadrant of the breast.

Mutation: An alteration of the genetic code.

Mutator genes: Abnormal genes that accelerate the production of oncogenes or defective tumor suppressor genes.

N

Necrosis: Dead tissue.

Needle biopsy: Removal and examination of a sample of tissue or fluid from the breast using a needle.

New primary: A new cancer that generally happens many years later and in an entirely different area of the breast.

Nipple: The small raised area in the center of the breast through which milk can flow to the outside.

Nipple-sparing mastectomy: The surgeon performs a mastectomy where the breast tissue is removed but the skin and nipple areolar complex are preserved. This technique is ideal for patients with small peripheral tumors or those high risk patients considering prophylactic mastectomy.

Nuclear grade: Evaluation of the size and shape of the nucleus in tumor cells and the percentage of tumor cells that are in the process of dividing or growing. Cancers with low nuclear grade grow and spread less quickly than cancers with high nuclear grade.

Nuclear magnetic resonance (NMRI or MRI): Imaging technique using a powerful magnet to transmit radio waves through the body to create detailed pictures of areas inside the body.

O

Oncogene: A gene that has mutated from the normal gene in cell growth.

Oncogene production: The production of proteins, leading to too much growth, such as cell division and invasion.

Oncologist: A physician who specializes in treating cancer.

Oncology: Study of cancer.

Oncotype DX breast cancer assay: This test is an analysis of twenty-one genetic markers that researchers consider important in predicting breast cancer behavior.

Oophorectomy: Surgical removal of the ovaries.

Osteoporosis: A marked decrease in bone density and mass, causing bones to weaken.

Ovarian ablation: Surgery, radiation or drug therapy used to stop the functioning of the ovaries.

P

p53 gene: A tumor suppressor gene that normally inhibits tumor growth.

Palpation: An examination procedure using the hands to press on the surface of the body to feel the tissues underneath.

Papillary: A non-invasive type of ductal cancer that does not spread and tends to be slow-growing.

Partial breast irradiation: Radiation just to the bed of the tumor rather than to the whole breast.

Pathologist: Doctor who performs many microscopic tests on tissue to determine the type, extent, and aggressiveness of cancer.

Pathology: The study of disease through the microscopic examination of body tissues and organs.

Pectoralis major: Muscle that lies under the breast.

Pedicle flap surgery: Surgery which involves removing muscle, skin, and fat from your donor site (the abdomen or back) but leaves the blood vessels attached during the transfer to the breast area. The tissue that has been removed is transferred underneath the skin, through a tunnel to the breast area while retaining its original blood supply.

Perforator flap surgery: A surgery which involves removing only skin, fat, and smaller blood vessels (perforators) from the donor site, leaving the underlying muscle intact. The donor tissue is transferred to the breast area and reattached using microsurgery.

Pituitary down-regulators: Drugs that reduce the production of estrogen stimulating hormones by the brain and may be given to pre-menopausal women.

Pituitary gland: The main gland located in the brain that produces hormones that control other glands in the body and body functions, especially growth.

Plastic surgeon: Doctor who will perform your reconstructive surgery if you choose to pursue it.

Platelet: A cell formed by the bone marrow and circulating in the blood that helps wounds heal and prevents bleeding by forming blood clots.

Port or Port-a-cath: A device surgically implanted under the skin that enters a large blood vessel and is used to deliver medication, chemotherapy, blood products and also is used to obtain blood samples.

Position emission tomography (PET) scan: This is procedure that involves injecting a small amount of radioactive glucose (sugar) into the bloodstream and then using a scanner to see if the cancer has spread to other areas of the body.

Post-menopausal: The time after menopause has occurred when menstruation has stopped permanently.

Pre-menopausal: The time before menopause.

Progesterone: Hormone that is released by the ovaries during each menstrual cycle to help prepare a woman's body for pregnancy and breastfeeding.

Prognosis: Expected or probable outcome of a disease; the chance of recovery or recurrence.

Prosthesis: Artificial substitute for an absent part of the body, such as breast prosthesis.

Protein: Formed from amino acids, this is the building block of life.

Protocol: Research designed to answer a hypothesis.

Psychologist: Specialist who can help with emotional responses before, during, and after treatments.

Q

Quadrantectomy: Surgical removal of the area of the breast (approximately one quarter) containing cancer.

R

Rad: A unit of absorbed radiation. One chest x-ray equals 1/10 of a rad.

Radiation oncologist: A physician specifically trained in the use of radiation to treat cancer.

Radiation therapy: Treatment with high energy x-rays to destroy cancer cells.

Radiation therapists: The technicians who operate the machines and administer therapy.

Radiation therapy or radiotherapy: The use of high-energy radiation from x-rays, gamma rays, neutrons, protons, and other sources to kill cancer cells and shrink tumors.

Radiologist: A physician who specializes in diagnoses of diseases by the use of x-rays.

Recurrence or recurrent cancer: Cancer that has come back after treatment is completed.

Regional recurrence: Cancer that has returned to lymph nodes.

Relapse: The appearance of cancer after a disease-free period.

Relative risk reduction: Is used to compare risks between two groups. It is the number that tells how different treatments, such as having radiation therapy, can change risk as compared to not having radiation therapy.

Remission: Disappearance of detectable disease.

Risk factors: Anything that increases an individual's chances of getting a disease such as cancer.

Risk reduction: Techniques used to reduce one's chances of getting a certain cancer.

S

Sarcoma: Cancer arising in the connective tissue.

Scleroderma: An autoimmune disease that involves thickening of the skin and difficulty swallowing, among other symptoms.

Secondary site: A second site in which cancer is found. Example: cancer in the lymph nodes near the breast is a secondary site.

Secondary tumor: A tumor that develops as a result of metastasis or spreads beyond the original cancer.

Segmental mastectomy: A procedure where the surgeon removes the tumor along with a larger area of tissue around the tumor and possibly the overlying skin. A portion of the lining of the chest wall muscle and skin may also be removed. Lymph nodes may or may not be removed by a separate incision.

Sentinel node biopsy: A procedure that involves the removal and examination of the first nodes (sentinel) to which the cancer cells are likely to have spread from the primary tumor.

SERM: Selective estrogen receptor modulator: a drug that acts like estrogen on some tissues but blocks estrogen on other tissues. Tamoxifen and raloxifene are SERMs.

Seroma: A pocket of fluid that sometimes develops in the body after surgery.

Side effect: Unintentional or undesirable secondary effect of treatment.

Skin-sparing mastectomy: The surgeon removes the breast tissue around the areola, nipple, and possibly lymph nodes. The excess skin and covering of the pectoral muscle is saved (spared) and used in the reconstruction of the breast. This type of surgery can be performed with either a modified radical or simple mastectomy.

Solid: A non-invasive type of cancer that tends to be slow-growing.

S phase fraction: Measures how many cells are dividing at a time; if it is high it is thought to indicate an aggressive tumor.

SPoT-Light Her-2 CISH (Subtraction Probe Technology Chromogenic In Situ Hybridization) test: A test that shows if there are too many copies of the HER-2/neu gene in the cancer cells.

Stage: Refers to the extent of cancer in the body. The TNM system looks at three elements when determining the stage of the cancer; the size of the tumor (T), whether lymph nodes are involved (N), and whether the cancer has spread beyond the breast to other sites of the body, metastasized (M).

Stereotactic needle biopsy: A biopsy done while the breast is compressed under mammography. A series of pictures locate the lesion and a radiologist enters information into a computer. The computer calculates information and positions a needle to remove the finding.

Stroma: The fatty tissue and connective tissue surrounding the ducts and lobules, blood vessels, and lymphatic vessels.

Surgeon: A doctor who removes or repairs a part of the body by operating.

Surgery: A local therapy or operational procedure to remove or repair a part of the body or to find out whether disease is present in an area.

Systemic treatment: Treatment involving substances that travel through the whole body, usually using drugs.

T

Tamoxifen: A drug that stops estrogen from binding to its receptor.

Targeted therapy: Treatment used to stimulate or restore the ability of the immune system to fight cancer, infections, and other diseases.

Taxanes: Drugs that prevent cancer cells from dividing.

Three-Dimensional Mammography: Also known as tomosynthesis is a type of mammogram that produces a 3D image of the breast and gives doctors a clearer view through the overlapping structures of breast tissue.

Tissue: A group or layer of similar cells that work together to perform a specific function.

Total or simple mastectomy: A procedure where the surgeon removes all of the breast tissue, the nipple, and areola, however, the pectoral muscle is not involved. Some of the lymph nodes under the arm may be removed.

Triple negative breast cancer: Describes breast cancer cells that do not have estrogen receptors, progesterone receptors, or large amounts of HER-2/neu protein.

Tumor: Abnormal mass of tissue. A tumor can be either benign or malignant.

Tumor markers: Hormones, proteins, or parts of proteins that are made by the tumor or by the body in response to the tumor.

Tumor suppressor gene: A gene that prevents cells from growing if they have a mutation.

U

Ultrasound examination: The use of high-frequency sound waves to form a picture of tissues inside the body.

Ultrasound guided biopsy: The use of ultrasound to guide a biopsy needle to obtain samples of tissue for analysis by a pathologist.

V

Vacuum-assisted breast biopsy (Mammotone): A procedure in which a tissue sample is removed using gentle vacuum suction and a small rotating knife within a probe.

Sources:

American Cancer Society

BreastCancer.org

Dictionary of Cancer Terms, National Cancer Institute: www.cancer.gov/dictionary

Bibliography

"Breast Cancer." Dr. Susan Love Research Foundation. Web. Oct.-Nov. 2010. <http://www.dslrf.org/breastcancer/content.asp?L2=4>.

ACSM | For the Exercise Sciences and Clinical Sports Medicine. Web. 17 Dec. 2010. <http://www.acsm.org/>.

American Cancer Society: Information and Resources for Cancer: Breast, Colon, Prostate, Lung and Other Forms. Web. Sept.-Oct. 2010. <http://www.cancer.org/>.

Bonner, Dede. *The 10 Best Questions for Surviving Breast Cancer*. First ed. New York: Fireside, 2008. Print.

"Breast Cancer: How Your Mind Can Help Your Body." American Psychological Association (APA). Web. Fall 2010. <http://www.apa.org/helpcenter/breast-cancer.aspx>.

"Breast Cancer in Men." American Cancer Society: Information and Resources for Cancer: Breast, Colon, Prostate, Lung and Other Forms. Web. 9 Nov. 2010. <http://www.cancer.org/Cancer/BreastCancerinMen/index>.

"Breast Cancer." RadiologyInfo–The Radiology Information Resource for Patients. Web. Jan. 2010. <http://www.radiologyinfo.org/en/info.cfm?pg=breastcancer>.

"Breast Cancer Recurrence." WebMD–Better Information. Better Health. Web. 4 Jan. 2011. <http://www.webmd.com/breast-cancer/guide/checking-for-recurrence>.

"Breast Cancer Treatment & Side Effects." BreastCancer.org–Breast Cancer Treatment Information and Pictures. Web. Oct.-Nov. 2010. <http://www.breastcancer.org/treatment/>.

"Breast Reconstruction After Mastectomy." American Cancer Society: Information and Resources for Cancer: Breast, Colon, Prostate, Lung and Other Forms. Web. Nov.-Dec. 2010. <http://www.cancer.org/Cancer/BreastCancer/MoreInformation/BreastReconstructionAfterMastectomy/index>.

"Breast Reconstruction Surgery–MD Anderson Cancer Center." Cancer Treatment and Cancer Research–MD Anderson Cancer Center. Web. Dec. 2010. <http://www.mdanderson.org/patient-and-cancer-information/cancer-information/cancer-topics/cancer-treatment/breast-reconstruction/index.html>.

Cancer Resources from OncoLink | Treatment, Research, Coping, Clinical Trials, Prevention. Web. 14 Nov. 2010. <http://www.oncolink.org/index.cfm>.

Cancer Support Community–Home. Web. 3 Sept. 2010. <http://www.thewellnesscommunity.org/>.

Cargiver.org. Web. 22 Nov. 2010. <http://cargiver.org>.

Carvalho, Lucia Giuggio., and J. A. Stewart. *The Everything Health Guide to Living with Breast Cancer: an Accessible and Comprehensive Resource for Women*. Avon, MA: Adams Media, 2009. Print.

Chan, David. *Breast Cancer: Real Questions, Real Answers*. New York: Marlowe &, 2006. Print.

Cohen, Deborah A., and Robert M. Gelfand. *Just Get Me through This: A Practical Guide to Coping with Breast Cancer*. New York: Kensington, 2003. Print.

"Disability Rights Legal Center–Protecting the Possibilities DisabilityRightsLegalCenter.org: About DRLC." Disability Rights Legal Center–Protecting the Possibilities. Web. Dec. 2010. <https://www.disabilityrightslegalcenter.org/about/cancerlegalresource.cfm>.

"Dictionary of Cancer Terms–National Cancer Institute." Comprehensive Cancer Information–National Cancer Institute. Web. Fall 2010. <http://www.cancer.gov/dictionary>.

Famous Quotes at BrainyQuote. Web. Winter 2010. <http://www.brainyquote.com/>.

"Fertility, Pregnancy, Adoption." BreastCancer.org–Breast Cancer Treatment Information and Pictures. Web. 20 Apr. 2011. <http://www.breastcancer.org/tips/fert_preg_adopt/>.

"For Patients | Journey Forward." Journey Forward | Journey Forward. Web. 26 Jan. 2011. <http://journeyforward.org/patients/patients>.

Hirshaut, Yashar, and Peter I. Pressman. *Breast Cancer: the Complete Guide*. New York: Bantam, 2008. Print.

"Hormone Therapy." American Cancer Society: Information and Resources for Cancer: Breast, Colon, Prostate, Lung and Other Forms. Web. 6 Mar. 2011. <http://www.cancer.org/Cancer/BreastCancer/DetailedGuide/breast-cancer-treating-hormone-therapy>.

Love, Susan M., and Karen Lindsey. *Dr. Susan Love's Breast Book*. Cambridge: Da Capo, 2010. Print.

Miller, Kenneth D. *Choices in Breast Cancer Treatment: Medical Specialists and Cancer Survivors Tell You What You Need to Know*. Baltimore: Johns Hopkins UP, 2008. Print.

National Center for Complementary and Alternative Medicine [NCCAM]–Nccam.nih.gov Home Page. Web. 14 Feb. 2011. <http://nccam.nih.gov/>.

The National Lymphedema Network–Web. 6 Nov. 2010. <http://www.lymphnet.org/>.

NCCS National Coalition for Cancer Survivorship. Web. Jan. 2011. <http://www.canceradvocacy.org/>.

National Institutes of Health (NIH). Web. Sept.–Oct. 2010. <http://nih.gov/>.

"Office of Cancer Complementary and Alternative Medicine (OCCAM)." Comprehensive Cancer Information - National Cancer Institute. Web. 10 Feb. 2011. <http://www.cancer.gov/cam/>.

Patient Advocate Foundation: 1-800-532-5274. Web. 12 Dec. 2010. <http://www.patientadvocate.org/>.

Shockney, Lillie. *Johns Hopkins Medicine Patients' Guide to Breast Cancer*. Sudbury, MA: Jones and Bartlett, 2010. Print.

"Sloan-Kettering–Diagnosis & Treatment at Memorial Sloan-Kettering: Systemic Therapy." Sloan-Kettering–Memorial Sloan-Kettering Cancer Center. Web. Fall 2010. <http://www.mskcc.

org/mskcc/html/2380.cfm>.

"Susan G. Komen for the Cure | Understanding Breast Cancer | After Treatment | After Treatment." Susan G. Komen for the Cure. Web. Jan. 2011. <http://ww5.komen.org/BreastCancer/aftertreatment.html>.

"Susan G. Komen for the Cure | Understanding Breast Cancer | Treatment | Treatment." Susan G. Komen for the Cure. Web. Sept.-Oct. 2011. <http://ww5.komen.org/BreastCancer/Treatment.html>.

Susan G. Komen for the Cure. Web. Jan.-Feb. 2010. <http://ww5.komen.org/>.

"Targeted Therapies Tutorials–National Cancer Institute." Comprehensive Cancer Information–National Cancer Institute. Web. 18 Nov. 2010. <http://www.cancer.gov/cancertopics/understandingcancer/targetedtherapies>.

"Types of Breast Reconstruction." American Cancer Society: Information and Resources for Cancer: Breast, Colon, Prostate, Lung and Other Forms. Web. Winter 2011. <http://www.cancer.org/Cancer/BreastCancer/MoreInformation/BreastReconstructionAfterMastectomy/breast-reconstruction-after-mastectomy-types-of-br-recon>.

Welcome to AdvancedBC.org | AdvancedBC.org. Web. Feb. 2011. <http://www.advancedbc.org/>.

Welcome to Young Survival Coalition: Young Women Facing Breast Cancer Together. Web. Fall 2010. <http://www.youngsurvival.org/>.

Index

> *For myself I am an optimist—it does not seem to be much use being anything else.*
>
> *- Winston Churchill*

Afterword

Life is good. Every day I am reminded of this. I am healthy, happy, and filled with gratitude. Since my initial diagnosis I've set and accomplished many personal goals, including writing this book. My first intention was to create a tool to help myself and others successfully navigate a breast cancer diagnosis. I feel I have achieved this and hope you do, too. My second intention is to continue to pay it forward by donating a portion of all profits from this book to help fund breast cancer research.

My thoughts and well wishes are with you and your families. I couldn't agree more with a fellow survivor:

"I had breast cancer, breast cancer didn't have me."

-Susan B.

Thank you for buying a copy of *Diagnosis: Breast Cancer—The Best Action Plan for Navigating Your Journey*. I'd love to hear how you are doing. I'm also interested in how this book has helped you, so please feel free to contact me and share your thoughts. I'd really appreciate it.

email: Cara@workoutcancer.com
Facebook: www.facebook.com/DiagnosisBC
Twitter: @CancerNavig8tor
Linked In: Cara Novy-Bennewitz

Thanks!

Cara

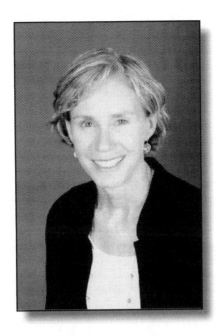

Cara Novy-Bennewitz is a Medical Ambassador for the American Cancer Society, a Certified Cancer Exercise Specialist, a Certified Health and Fitness Instructor by the American College of Sports Medicine, and an Exercise Physiologist. She is a graduate of Drake University and has spent her entire career specializing in health, wellness, and preventive medicine. She has been a personal trainer for over 15 years, is currently the Wellness Consultant for the Evanston Police Department, and is the head of Physical Education for School District 68.

Cara is a distance runner, who eats healthy, exercises regularly, and believes in enjoying life. She is also a breast cancer survivor, being unexpectedly diagnosed in her early 40s with a young child. She mistakenly thought the odds were in her favor of avoiding cancer given her healthy lifestyle choices and no family history of breast cancer. As a seasoned educator and presenter, Cara hopes to empower patients and their loved ones throughout their breast cancer journeys.

When not coaching people on health and wellness Cara is often doing something active with her family, watching movies, or reading a book. Her husband likes to joke that reading is a form of birth control—if she's reading a good book, he knows to stay away!